Play Therapy:

A Non-directive Approach for Children and Adolescents

!7

Play Therapy
A Non-directive Approach for Children and Adolescents

KATE WILSON
BA (Oxon), Dip.SWK (Sussex)
Lecturer in Social Work at the University of Hull and
Director of the University's post-qualifying course in child
protection.

PAULA KENDRICK
BA (Hons), Dip.Ed, CQSW
College Counsellor, Wyke Sixth Form College, Hull;
formerly Project Leader, Child Sexual Abuse Unit,
Humberside Social Services.

VIRGINIA RYAN
BA, summa cum laude, PhD
Child psychologist, lecturing in child protection and child
development at the University of Hull.

Baillière Tindall

LONDON · PHILADELPHIA · SYDNEY · TOKYO · TORONTO

Baillière Tindall

24–28 Oval Road
London NW1 7DX, UK

The Curtis Center,
Independence Square West,
Philadelphia, PA 19106–3399, USA

55 Homer Avenue
Toronto, Ontario M8Z 4X6, Canada

Harcourt Brace Jovanovich Group
(Australia) Pty Ltd.,
30–52 Smidmore St,
Marrickville, NSW 2204, Australia

Harcourt Brace Jovanovich (Japan) Inc.,
Ichibancho Central Building,
22–1 Ichibancho
Chiyoda-ku, Tokyo 102, Japan

This book is printed on acid-free paper

ISBN 0–7020–1487–7

A catalogue record for this book is available from The British Library

Typeset by J&L Composition Ltd, Filey, North Yorkshire, UK.
Printed in Great Britain by Mackays of Chatham PLC,
Chatham, Kent, UK.

The cover illustration is adapted from a painting given by a child with whom one of the authors worked.

Plates 1–6 were kindly supplied by the University of Hull Photographic & Copy Service, Brynmor Jones Library ©.

Contents

Preface

Our greatest hope for this book is that it will be of practical use and that it will assist professionals in providing effective help for the troubled children with whom they work.

We aim to provide a comprehensive introduction to non-directive play therapy and to demonstrate that this is both a viable and robust method of working with emotionally damaged children. Clearly, we also wish to see the approach practised more widely, so that it may be more generally available in the treatment of children. We hope that the book will serve as a means of achieving this.

In organizing the book, we needed to take into account a number of factors. First, we hoped to reach a wide audience. Although we were aware that every professional needs to bear in mind issues of role, organizational context, resources, and the statutory and legal requirements of the work, we also recognized that these concerns would vary in their degree of urgency for different professionals. We have therefore tried when addressing these issues to acknowledge this diversity in professional role.

Equally, we have wanted the book to be useful to both experienced and inexperienced practitioners and hope that the material in it will be sufficiently challenging to the former, while at the same time providing detailed guidance for the beginning therapist. (The book cannot, however, be a substitute for training, and we would emphasize here, as we do again in the text, the importance of being supervised when undertaking therapeutic work.)

We have sought to clarify some of the confusions which in our experience currently surround the place of therapy in the child protection process, and explore this in some detail in Chapter 1, where we set non-directive play therapy in its historical and contemporary context and compare it with other past and current therapeutic approaches.

For reasons which we touch on in Chapter 1, non-directive play therapy is often described in a somewhat a-theoretical manner. Nonetheless, the practitioner does need to be able to set play therapy in a theoretical framework: indeed, to use Lewin's oft-quoted phrase, 'there is nothing so practical as a good theory', and if the book is to achieve its practical purpose, then practitioners require theoretical frameworks and concepts in order to make sense of the process of therapy, guide their interventions, and retrieve errors.

In Chapter 2, therefore, we develop our theoretical understanding of play, and of the effectiveness of play therapy, within a general framework of mental development. This framework provides the basis for our later discussions about the process of intervention.

Planning decisions and tasks are considered in detail in Chapter 3, and this is followed by an illustrative account of play therapy with a six-year-old girl, and a consideration of specific issues that arise in working with children in middle childhood and adolescence. We then include a chapter on working with children who have been sexually abused, considering that this group of children pose particular problems for the therapist.

We conclude by considering four issues, namely the reflection of feelings, limit setting, responding to disclosures within therapy and court work, which in our experience of teaching non-directive play therapy require particular exploration. All those currently concerned with abused children must be conscious of the legal and statutory framework to their work and issues arising from undertaking therapy in a legal context are therefore considered in this final chapter in some detail.

We have changed the names and some of the details concerning the children to whom we refer in order to safeguard their privacy. Since all the authors are women, it seemed simplest to adopt 'she' for the therapist and 'he' for the child, although for the latter, where it does not seem to interrupt the flow of the text, we have said 'he or she'. We had some difficulty in deciding between 'practitioner', 'worker' and 'therapist', being aware that different professional groups would be likely to feel more comfortable with different terminology. On the whole we use the term therapist, as it most accurately reflects the therapeutic nature of non-directive play therapy.

Finally, we acknowledge with gratitude the support of our families during the writing of this book and, in particular, Dan's valiant efforts with our wordprocessor. We are grateful to our colleague, John Mullins, and to our students for allowing us to use some of their case material. We also thank our main typist, Mary Squires, and Sarah Smith, Gill Robinson and Penny Robinson of Baillière Tindall for their advice and encouragement. Above all, we are indebted to the children with whom we have worked and to whom this book is dedicated.

1

Introduction

The purpose of this book is to provide an introduction to a particular approach to helping children and adolescents, many although not all of whom may have been abused, either physically, emotionally or sexually. It is intended for all those who, through their professional role, may be asked to work directly with emotionally damaged children. Although we shall pay particular attention to the issues and dilemmas which we know confront practitioners working with children within a statutory framework, we hope that what we describe will also be of interest to professionals in related settings such as psychologists and specialist health care professionals.

The approach to working with children and adolescents described in the book is based on one particular way of working: that of non-directive counselling or play therapy. Briefly expressed, the approach involves a special one-to-one relationship, where the therapist creates a safe and trusting climate in which the individual is free, if he chooses to do so, to express and explore some of his feelings. These may be communicated either directly (as Berry, 1978, describes it, "in words accurately or obliquely phrased"), or indirectly through behaviour and play. The task of the therapist is to listen, understand and respond to these communications in such a way as to help the individual towards a greater awareness of feelings, which when expressed and experienced in an accepting relationship lose much of their negative power. Berry, writing about communication with children within this relationship, suggests that

It can bring great relief for a child to risk being in touch with his feelings, which lose some of their negative influence once they reach the light of day, when they are expressed and contained without any terrible repercussions. So the child who is given opportunities to communicate tends to gain more control

1

over his own behaviour and to feel less at the mercy of haphazard events. He is less isolated; his life begins to have more coherence, pattern and meaning. (1978: 181)

The emphasis in the work is thus on enabling the individual to move from a sense of being at the mercy of hidden feelings to gaining some mastery over them.

This therapeutic approach is based on the principles of non-directive psychotherapy developed by Rogers. Most readers will be familiar with these, and will have incorporated some of them into their practice. Many, too, will be familiar with the work of Axline, who most famously in **Dibs: In Search of Self** (1946) and subsequently in **Play Therapy** (1947) describes an approach to working with children which is in essence an extension of Rogerian psychotherapy, but takes account of the fact that play is 'the child's natural medium for self-expression'. (1947: 16) The underlying philosophy of the approach is that there exists in all human beings a drive for self-realization, which motivates both children and adults. The assumption is that given the opportunity to express themselves freely, children will play through their conflicts and arrive at a solution to them. It is with Axline's approach to play therapy, adapted and modified to take account of the different practice requirements of the British context, and other clinical developments which have taken place since she first developed it, that we are concerned here.

We consider that a book on therapeutic interventions with children is timely. Much public and professional concern over the past decade or so has been directed towards ensuring that professionals whose work brings them into direct contact with children are able to recognize situations when abuse is occurring, and know how to take the appropriate steps, legal or otherwise, to protect children from further abuse. Public attention, and as a consequence of this, major shifts in policy and in practice, have focused on the need to protect children who have been identified as being at risk of abuse. That this has occurred largely as a result of public inquiries set up in the wake of the tragic deaths of children has had certain consequences for the process of intervention: it has tended to focus attention on the attempt to understand why these tragedies occurred; more particularly, since many of the inquiries concerned children who died at a time when a variety of professionals were actively involved with them and their families, on making sense of how it was that those with professional responsibility for the children failed to perceive what was happening and to intervene to protect them. Thus much of the discussion has been directed towards detection, assessment, and the proper and effective communication of information between professionals and to a lesser extent parents, about the children concerned.

Even in the one major public inquiry not involving the death of a child (Butler-Sloss, 1988), the point of departure was a concern to establish whether or not in removing the children concerned from their parents, the authorities had acted appropriately or otherwise. Thus, the reasons why the inquiries were set up, and their terms of reference, have produced almost inevitably a concentration on establishing a knowledge base in relation to risk assessment (see, for example, Brent, 1985) and on developing procedures which would limit the possibility of the recurrence of serious and life-threatening mistakes.

Furthermore, the quasi-legalistic manner in which the inquiries have been conducted has tended to militate against detailed discussion of what, if any, therapeutic work was being undertaken with the children. This is of course partly because of the terms of reference with which they were set up but also perhaps because of the more individualistic nature of therapy and the difficulty of describing it succinctly to those conducting the investigation. The Cleveland Report acknowledges the distinction between investigative and therapeutic work, and emphasizes the fact that the two processes should not be confused; this apart, virtually no reference is made to therapeutic work in the now extensive documentation of child abuse intervention.

However, along with greater confidence in the existence of appropriate procedures must come a greater awareness of their fallibility and their limitations – an acknowledgement that however well, broadly speaking, procedures are adhered to, they may in fact do little to address the knottier problems surrounding the abuse of children. Equally there has been an increasing recognition of the therapeutic needs of the child and of the fact that action to protect the child does not necessarily address the suffering which may be consequent on the abuse. The Children Act, with its emphasis on partner-ship, and its recognition that practitioners in statutory agencies will increasingly be involved in purchasing specific services for their clients, seems likely to provide further encouragement for the provision of therapeutic interventions (James and Wilson, 1991).

We hope that a book which addresses the problem of how to help in terms which go beyond investigation, diagnosis, assessment and planning will redress a balance which has up to now tended to concentrate on guidelines and procedures and paid less attention to work with the abused, neglected or troubled child.

Our second and perhaps principal purpose in writing this book is that there seems to us an absence of any book which provides a detailed practice guide to an approach to therapeutic work which is both effective and accessible. We shall demonstrate that non-directive play therapy is a way of working which is ethically sound, and which, because it ensures that the child is respected, listened to, and not intruded upon, is likely to be particularly acceptable to the courts.

We recognize in writing about one particular method of working that we are to some extent breaking with tradition. Practitioners in Britain have by custom and perhaps by inclination tended to draw selectively on theory rather than adhering strictly to one conceptual approach to intervention. This we would regard as being the case in other therapeutic work, for example with marital intervention or with family therapy as much as in work with children. In some ways, this eclecticism may be seen as a strength, in that it permits a greater creative innovation than may be possible in countries such as the United States or Germany where there is more emphasis on schools and training in one method of intervention. It does, however, in our view have certain drawbacks: it is arguably easier to develop and modify a therapeutic approach when one has been thoroughly trained in it. Such training is very hard to come by in this country. It may also mean that such training and practice guides as exist are in fact difficult to learn from, just because they represent a collection of ideas and precepts about practice without any unifying theory. This for example we consider to be the limitation of two recent books on direct work with children (Aldgate and Simmonds, 1988; Doyle, 1990). Although they offer relevant advice and give a broad overview of work with children, their usefulness as practice guides is limited, either because they attempt, as in the case of Doyle, to consider a broad range of therapies in a short amount of space, or because as in the case of Aldgate and Simmonds, the book is an edited one, with no single identifiable approach to intervention.

One further justification, if one is needed, for the book is that it is apparent from our involvement in training in child therapy and in social work practice that there is a good deal of confusion over the purpose and application of play therapy as opposed to play related interventions such as assessments or validation interviews. These may frequently use play as a means of assisting the communication between child and practitioner, and may well, if conducted with sensitivity, have therapeutic value for the child. However, their purpose and method of intervention is very different from that of sustained therapeutic work, and needs to be distinguished from it.

In order to clarify this distinction, and also to place non-directive play therapy in the historical context of its development alongside other child psychotherapies, in the first half of this chapter we shall examine what seem to us to be the principal developments in the field of working therapeutically with children, reviewing the commonalities between them, together with their distinguishing features. In the following section, we consider the historical context in which non-directive play therapy has developed and the broad principles and skills of the approach.

| S E C T I O N   O N E |

DIFFERENT APPROACHES TO CHILD PSYCHOTHERAPY

Any attempt at classifying therapeutic approaches must take into account the fact that although some models are distinctive and have developed their own skills and techniques which are not readily interchangeable with those from other models, this is not necessarily the case and that some methods have clearly developed by borrowing from other treatment modalities. Moreover, while some, such as psychoanalytic therapies, are based on clearly formulated theoretical principles with organized training and practice implementation, others, such as structured play therapy, are more loosely defined and in some respects appear to have developed in an ad hoc and pragmatic manner. There is a risk therefore that a classification may suggest that the distinctions between the approaches are more clear-cut than in fact they are, and this caveat should be borne in mind in what follows.

We have tried, within the discussion, to identify those features of each model which appear most significant, focusing particularly on the issue of the purpose and style of the interventions made by the therapist and the principles on which they are based.

PSYCHOANALYTIC PLAY THERAPY

We begin here, because although this approach to therapy is currently used comparatively rarely with children, historically it is significant in that the work of Freud, Klein and Anna Freud provided a stimulus to developments elsewhere in the therapeutic use of play.

Although Freud himself worked predominantly with adults, his analysis of little Hans (with the father as therapist) and his observations on the meaning of children's play pointed the way to the later development by Klein and Anna Freud of child psychoanalysis. His writing on children's play reflects an intuitive grasp of its significance, and although he did not develop these ideas, they are worth quoting both for the observations themselves, and for their contribution to later thought:

The child's best loved and most absorbing occupation is play. Perhaps we may say that every child at play behaves like an imaginative writer, in that he creates a world of his own or, more truly, he arranges the things of his world and orders it in a new way that pleases him better. It would be incorrect to say that he does not take his world seriously; on the contrary, he takes his play very seriously and expends a great deal of emotion on it. The opposite of play is not serious occupation, but reality. Notwithstanding the large affective cathexis of his play world, the child distinguishes it perfectly from reality; only he likes to borrow the objects and circumstances that he imagines from the tangible and real world. It is only this linking of it to reality that still distinguishes a child's 'play' from 'daydreaming'. (Freud, 1974: 173–174)

Klein and Anna Freud, working in Vienna and London in the 1920s and 1930s, made a lasting contribution to the development of play therapy. Both believed many childhood psychiatric disorders to be the result of unconscious conflicts, and held that these would be resolved, and the child's ego strengthened, by bringing these unconscious elements to consciousness through the interpretation of the child's play and dreams by the therapist. Both considered insight to be an essential part of resolution, and that it does not occur without a process of 'working through'.

In interaction with the therapist, in play or words, the child repeatedly displays his basic conflicts . . . interpretation of his feelings, thoughts and motives fosters mastery of conflicts and maturation. (Wolff, 1986: 225)

The child's play was seen to take the place, in analysis, of the adult's free association; like the latter, it is free from the censorship of reality. The prime task of the child analyst is therefore to understand and interpret the symbolic content of the child's play. To this end Klein in particular equipped the therapy room with a range of play materials, representational figures and non-mechanical toys designed to stimulate and foster the child's imaginative play.

Although there are important differences between Klein and Anna Freud (principally concerning the nature of the relationship between therapist and child, and the extent of the interpretation of the child's verbal and non-verbal communications), their contribution to the development of understanding and working with children is undoubted, and others working with children have drawn on their methods and insights. However, as with adult psychoanalysis, child psychoanalysis is highly specialized and time-consuming, demanding as it does intervention over a number of years. It is therefore possible for writers such as Marvasti, in his discussion of different forms of play therapy, to state firmly that "[this] modality of therapy . . . is indicated only in some neurotic children and is not appropriate therapy for a child with sexual trauma but no long-standing neurotic conflicts". (1989: 21)

On both sides of the Atlantic, this approach has therefore largely given way to what Wolff terms "psychoanalytically oriented psychotherapy", that is, approaches which draw on the same principles and techniques, but which are more focused, briefer, and whose aims are more circumscribed. In the development of this, the contribution of Winnicott has been significant.

OBJECT RELATIONS THERAPY

Winnicott, although trained as a Kleinian, worked within the British School of object-relations therapies (propounded, among others, by Fairbairn, Dicks and Bowlby) and developed his own influential, if idiosyncratic, approach to working with children. He saw play as central to the therapeutic experience, believing that children's play has direct continuity with what he described as an 'intermediate area' in adult experience, such as art and religion, where the strain of managing the transition between inner and outer reality is relatively unchallenged and therefore anxiety free. Play was in his view therefore the means whereby the child manages the transition between the inner world of the psyche and outer reality and thus "always on the theoretical line between the subjective and that which is objectively perceived". (Winnicott, 1988: 59)

Although working primarily with the material presented by the child in play, his approach may be classified as directive and interpretive: directive because the therapist may at times select the particular form of play as a means of communicating (for example, the famous squiggle game, in which therapist and child take turns to complete a picture from a line that the other has drawn, and then comment on what they have drawn); interpretive because the therapist, in responding to the child's play and dreams, articulates the link between the manifest behaviour and hidden, usually unconscious feelings. The systematic uncovering of unconscious material is thus the principal focus, but the material uncovered is circumscribed by limitations of the time available for therapy.

It is clear however from his writings and case examples, that Winnicott adopted a variety of approaches in working with children: sometimes seeing the child's play as mirroring the experience being described by the carer (usually the mother), and sometimes interpreting this to her, sometimes not; sometimes responding to the communication within its own terms and metaphor, without exploring its underlying symbolic meaning; sometimes interpreting and linking it to historical material; and so on. Winnicott's approach has at times much in common with non-directive play therapy, and indeed, in acknowledging that "psychotherapy of a deep-going kind may be done without interpretive work", he quotes Axline with approval (Winnicott, 1988: 59). Moreover, the ideas which he developed about the place of play in helping the child communicate and achieve mastery over his or her inner and outer reality provide insight into the therapeutic processes which we seek to explore.

Fascinating and often inspiring though his work is, however, the very invention and creativity which is its hallmark also make his methods sometimes seem elusive and difficult to follow or practise. We must therefore concur with Wolff's comment, who pointing out that Winnicott did not establish a 'school' or training programme of his own, concludes, "Whether other less intuitive therapists can use his methods as effectively remains in doubt." (Wolff, 1986: 227)

COGNITIVE–BEHAVIOURAL APPROACHES

These are based, as the reader will be aware, on a view of the personality which sees virtually all behaviour as learned and purposive: therapy is based on cognitive–behavioural understandings and is directive, in that it is the therapist who in conjunction with the client agrees the goals of intervention and sets up a programme of activity and response designed to give positive reinforcement to desirable behaviours and to extinguish those which are identified as undesirable. Although the therapist's focus and style of response is clearly different, it is, as a number of writers have demonstrated, possible to find common ground between those from the behaviourist and those from the psychodynamic school in their view of the therapeutic experience. Thus Truax and Carkhuff (1967) although writing about the therapeutic relationship from a Rogerian perspective, consider that at least some aspects of the interactions between client and worker can be conceptualized from a perspective of learning theory:

It might be tentatively proposed that these three 'therapeutic conditions' have their direct and indirect effects upon patient change in the following four modalities:

(1) They serve to reinforce positive aspects of the patient's self-concept.

(2) They serve to reinforce self-exploratory behaviour.

(3) They serve to extinguish anxiety or fear responses associated with specific cues.

(4) They serve to reinforce human relating, encountering or interacting, and to extinguish fear or avoidance learning associated with human relating. (quoted in Sutton, 1979: 52)

From a cognitive perspective, one might add a further function:

(5) They also allow inconsistencies of feeling, attitude and behaviour to be unravelled, and a fuller integration to emerge. (Sutton, 1979: 52)

However, despite these commonalities, behavioural approaches to work with children are distinctive in that the principles underlying these treatments are largely the same for children as for adults. In traditional behavioural intervention play-based activities are rarely used, helping techniques are often undertaken by the child's parents or teachers and may focus on the child's interaction with his environment. On these three counts therefore, behavioural approaches are distinct from other psychotherapeutic approaches which we consider here.

RELEASE THERAPY

This form of play therapy is directed towards helping a child who has experienced a particular painful or traumatic event to work through and gain mastery over the feelings engendered by it. The therapy is based on the psychoanalytic idea of repetition compulsion, where by re-enacting and re-experiencing a particular event, pent-up or blocked off feelings are released and eventually extinguished. Although the child is free to choose the kind of play he wishes, the play materials are limited and selected in order to encourage him to make use of those connected with the trauma.

This approach was developed in America by Levy (1938). It does however bear similarities, in the careful selection of specific play materials, to the 'World Technique' introduced by Lowenfeld at the London Institute of Child Psychology in the 1920s and currently used, in a modified version, by the Newsons at the Child Development Research Unit in Nottingham. The child is presented with trays filled with sand and using a range of miniature but realistic objects (people, houses, cars, trees, farm equipment and so on) is encouraged to create a three-dimensional picture – 'a world' in the sand. Lowenfeld would explain to the child that the way in which she played had a meaning which they would discover and explore together. Lowenfeld considered that the worlds created by the child frequently reflected facets of the child's problems, and that by commenting on the child's play the child could become aware of and clarify the confused emotions, experiences and sensations which she called 'non-verbal thinking'. Interpretations were withheld until the child reached 'emotional readiness'; at which point (if the interpretation was correct) the play would change and new themes would appear. (Lowenfeld, 1979)

Although there are elements in Lowenfeld's work which correspond to the non-directive approach, in that for much of the time the therapist's comments are descriptive and not interpretive, it is clearly based on psychoanalytic principles. The definite structure given to the therapy session and the encouragement to play in a particular way suggest that it has much in common with the therapeutic approach developed by Levy and derives from this tradition rather than from Rogers.

The Newsons' approach, while borrowing extensively from Lowenfeld, has closer links with non-directive play therapy. The model Newson describes (in press) uses a two-part therapy session, in which the therapist largely eschews interpretation: in the first part, the child is encouraged to make and play in a World, using specially selected play equipment; the second involves free-play, and the therapist tells the child that "he's 'the Boss' and she is there to help him in whatever he wants to play".

The underlying philosophy, which resembles that of non-directive play therapy, is that the child will select, and work on through play, issues which have meaning for him, and which may not be fully understood by the therapist; the therapist "facilitates the work that the child needs to do", rather than directing or interpreting it.

ABREACTIVE PLAY THERAPY

The abreactive approach to play therapy developed by Solomon (1938) also bears some similarity to the release therapy described earlier, in its identification of therapeutic goals, although not in its means of attaining them. In this country, a similar approach seems to have been adopted in some of their work with abused children by clinicians and social workers at the Great Ormond Street Hospital for Sick Children (see, for example, Stevens and Walsh, 1987: 286). The child is encouraged to act out negative emotions of fear, anger and hostility through play, and may be directly confronted or challenged to express them if he or she appears to be blocking, denying or using other mechanisms to defend against acknowledging the trauma. The principle of change on which this approach is based seems to be that re-experiencing the negative emotions surrounding the child's trauma produces an abreactive (cathartic) effect, particularly when these can be acted-out without producing a negative reaction from the therapist. Solomon also appears to suggest that in order to get in touch with these negative feelings and to be released from them, it is necessary to reproduce some of the feelings of trauma through the painful breaking down of defences.

There is some common ground between this approach and non-directive therapy in certain aspects of its understanding of how therapeutic change occurs, that is, the bringing to light, and the re-experiencing in the context of an uncritical relationship, of negative emotions. However, this approach is not compatible with the non-directive approach with its emphasis on going at the child's pace. Moreover, there are major differences in the view of the way in which re-experiencing painful feelings enables the child to be released from them. Although reliving them within the therapeutic session can undoubtedly be painful for the child, the emphasis in non-directive work is on enabling the child to feel in control of when and how defences are lowered and painful material addressed. By remaining in control, the child is encouraged to feel able to master frightening or negative emotions. If, as it appears, in abreactive therapy, these defences are breached by the therapist in order to re-enact the trauma, it is difficult to see how the child's trust and sense of self-reliance can be secured. It is also clearly imperative that the child has sufficient ego resources and support, and sufficient trust and confidence in the therapist for such confrontation to be undertaken safely, conditions which may well not pertain. Finally, the behaviours required of the therapist seem likely to encourage aggressive and over-intrusive interventions on the part of the therapist unless carefully and expertly supervised. For these reasons, we consider this approach inappropriate for most clinical settings.

STRUCTURED PLAY THERAPY

This approach has been principally developed by Oaklander (1978) working in a gestalt framework. In it the therapist uses a variety of techniques to guide the child directly or indirectly into areas of play which will enable child and therapist to work on a particular area of the child's experience, usually one which has previously been identified as problematic by another adult or by the therapist in an assessment interview. Techniques and play materials are varied, depending on the assessment of the problem, but may include such things as mutual story-telling (where the child is asked to tell a story, and the therapist then creates a responding story with the same characters and events but with healthier adaptations and conflict resolution); guided fantasy; the empty chair technique, and so on. Oaklander's work is clearly imaginative and inventive, and her ideas have been used and adapted by practitioners both here and in America (see, for example, Aldgate and Simmonds, 1988).

In this country, Redgrave among others has developed the use of what he calls 'focused play', seeing this as using therapist techniques which he calls 'directive', and distinguishing it from 'free- or non-focused play'. (1987: 25) Although he makes only passing reference to this distinction and does not explore the differences in any detail, it seems a valid one to make, and from the available literature it would appear that much of the play therapy undertaken in British settings shares many of the characteristics of Redgrave's structured, focused-play approach. Life-story work, or the techniques for use in 'anger Work' described by Owen and Curtis (1983) seem to fall into this category of structured play.

Redgrave describes, as an example of structured work, helping children who have bottled up anger to see that there are 'helpful and unhelpful ways of expressing anger' by drawing, activities or graphic illustrations using a steam engine to illustrate bottled up anger. Or in working with another child, Alexander,

I was interested in helping him to develop a conscience about kind and unkind behaviour in himself. So I used the idea of a pair of old fashioned scales ... Again I had a number of small cards, some with kind or helpful actions written on them, others with unhelpful or unkind actions and some left blank ... Alexander recognised an ongoing aim to bring the scales down on the righthand, 'positive', side over the weeks of using the scales. We had a score scale on this side but not on the negative side. (Redgrave, 1987: 93)

Many of these devices for helping children understand feelings and make sense of what has happened or is happening to them, can appropriately be incorporated into a non-directive approach, and we discuss their use in a later chapter. However, partly because the basis on which each technique is adopted is often unclear, particularly in Oaklander's writing, there is a danger that utilizing these techniques can encourage something of a shopping basket approach to working with children, selecting exercises or other devices haphazardly and often more in response to the practitioner's uncertainty about how to 'deal with' a particular problem than in response to an identified feeling or need on the part of the child. Moreover, some cognitive devices are, as we discuss in chapter 2, inappropriate for some, especially young, children.

PLAY-RELATED INTERVENTIONS

We consider here, finally, a whole range of play-related activities which have been developed in order to enable child and practitioner to communicate more effectively with each other about critical events. We recognize that interviews conducted for the purpose of making assessments, or in order to prepare the child for a critical life event such as a move to foster care may provide a therapeutic experience for the child. However, we want to make a distinction here between play therapies of the kind which we have been considering, where the intervention is sustained and the aim is to bring about some change in the child's functioning, and those interventions where the aim relates to a particular task identified by the practitioner. In the latter the aim is circumscribed, and by and large directed towards improving planning and decision-making and the impact of these interventions on the child.

Although a hard and fast distinction may in practice be difficult to sustain, some acknowledgement should be made of the differences between those interventions where play activities are used because they are seen as a medium in which the child may be more comfortable and can communicate more easily; and those where the child is encouraged to play with certain carefully selected play materials. In the latter, through the interpretation of the symbolic meaning of the child's play an assessment is made of the child's principal emotional conflicts, the existence of trauma and its impact on the child's personality and subsequent development.

Play-related communications

A number of practitioners (for example, Bray, verbal communication, Redgrave, 1987; Williamson, 1990) describe interventions where play materials are used to facilitate the communication between adult and child and to help the child's understanding of events. Thus, for example, many practitioners investigating an allegation of abuse may use a puppet animal, a telephone or play figures in a doll's house in the interview with the child. The underlying assumptions are that children can displace their emotions on to play materials, and may have less anxiety in communicating for example with a puppet than directly with an adult. Children are less verbal than adults, and particularly before a certain cognitive stage has been reached, find non-verbal means of com- municating more accessible. By playing, it is easier for the therapist to assess the child's level of understanding of a given situation.

Redgrave, for example, describes using a range of play-related activities when undertaking work with children where

in connection with the social and psychosocial situations involving the child we are ... exploring or trying to explain how things are. Many devices ... may be used for the purpose of helping the child to deal with social and psychosocial aspects of his life and present situation. The ecomap or sociogram is an obvious example. Sliders may also be used for this purpose ... It is quite easy to design 'special' devices or games for a particular child and then to find that these have a general use since many other children can be helped with the same device. (Redgrave, 1987: 91)

He describes for example work with a child Carl, where a decision had been taken to move from a foster home this one child out of a sibling group of three:

Before using the doll's house with Carl on his own, I read to him the cartoon story of Mint, the kitten ... This is about a kitten who, like most kittens, has to leave his first mum and then goes to live with a very nice lady, but has to move **again** .... After that I used two of the cardboard box rooms to represent two houses. With the cardboard cut-out figures I acted two or three small scenes, one of them taking place in the house that had no children and where the married couple were saying how much they wished they had a little boy. Eventually the cut-out child named Carl (all the others were given names different to the real family) went to live with the childless couple. Then the cut- out children made visits to each other's houses. By the time the end of the 'play' was reached the real Carl was talking quite easily about a real move. Remember, he was already unsettled in the family. (1987: 89)

This approach to communicating with children will, we judge, be familiar to a social work audience. We have quoted this example in some detail because we consider that the difference should be stressed between the use of play in play therapy and in activities such as these which are used by an adult to explain, clarify, prepare or for other purposes, work on an area which the adult has identified as one of concern.

Play diagnosis and assessment

Play diagnosis has been defined by Marvasti as "a technique to enable a child to reveal internal conflicts, fantasies, wishes and perceptions of the world ..." (1989: 1) Play materials are carefully selected in order to enable the practitioner to focus on significant events in a child's life, and to assess their impact on the child's personality and subsequent development. The use of play in diagnostic assessments is based on the idea that in play, a child may act out his true feelings with the help of certain of the main ego mechanisms of defence, most commonly projection, displacement and symbolization. The usual anxieties and constraints (for example about revealing anger towards a new sibling, or the disturbing and frightening actions of an adult) do not operate because the feelings are projected or displaced on to the play materials. Thus the activities are 'done' for example by dolls rather than the child and can be safely expressed. For example:

During the second play session, Jimmy arranged the family dolls inside the dollhouse. Then the mother doll brought a new puppy, which became the center of attention. Later a monster from outside came and kidnapped the new puppy. (Marvasti, 1989: 2)

The child's play can be seen to reflect his resentment at the arrival of a baby sister, and the anger which he feels, and the destructive impulses towards her, are displaced on to the monster. The child also uses symbolization, substituting a puppy for the baby sister.

What is also clear from this example is that the child at play is preoccupied generally with psychic reality, that is, his own perception of events, rather than objective reality. The child's psychic reality may, through wishfulness or fear, for example, be a distortion of objective reality. Thus, in this instance, the practitioner could comment with some confidence on the child's psychic reality, his perception of events; and from a balance of probability, might make a distinction between this and what was actually occurring in the child's environment. In terms of assessment as a prelude for therapeutic work with the child, the practitioner's primary concern is with identifying the child's wishes and feelings, and therefore establishing the basis in reality of the child's play is less crucial. However, much work with children involves the need to protect, and to plan for them. One of the practitioner's tasks therefore may be to interpret the child's play, understand its symbolic meaning and try and establish what in the child's perception of events has objective rather than subjective reality. (See chapter 7, section 4 for a fuller discussion of this, and the value of the non-directive approach as evidence of the child's own perception.)

It seems likely that the theory about play, and therefore the reasons for its use, are similar in play diagnosis and in the play-related interventions we describe above. Thus the practitioner who uses animal puppets with a child in an investigation of abuse does so partly at least because it will be less intimidating for a child to 'talk' through animals – that is, the constraints involved in a direct verbal exchange are lifted, and the child can displace feelings and actions on to the puppet. Play is also a means of addressing the limitations imposed by the younger child's limited verbal capacity and cognitive awareness. Thus before a child has reached the stage of what Piaget describes as 'formal operations', and becomes capable of abstract thought, it may be easier to use physical representations of things which are familiar (a tree to represent the past history of a family, for example) than words. Thus the use of play is based on an understanding of it as an area free from constraints, and also on an assessment of the child's intellectual, emotional and cognitive development.

However, we want to retain the distinction between the two approaches which we have made in the above discussion, since play diagnosis as we have described it here makes greater use of the child's capacity for free play, and depends to a greater extent on the practitioner's observation, assessment and interpretation of the child's activity. To this extent, it is likely that, although play materials are carefully selected, the techniques used are less directive than in the play-related communications described above.

COMMONALITIES IN THESE APPROACHES

We have in this section highlighted the distinctions which are discernible in different approaches to working directly with children. We have tried to demonstrate that these distinctions arise partly out of a difference in the underlying purpose of the work. This is clearly the case in interviews under-taken for reasons of assessment, but also in those situations where the practitioner rather than the child has an identified purpose in conducting the interview. Some of the differences between approaches reflect a difference in belief about how change occurs (as with abreactive therapy), and there are evident differences in the extent to which therapists consider it necessary to acknowledge to the child the links between past and present, or to interpret to the child the symbolic meaning of his play. The role of insight in the approaches is therefore either indistinct or variable. However, in those therapies which involve work with the child alone some similarities of principles and goals of treatment are discernible (see also Marvasti, 1989.) (We exclude here first those approaches whose purposes are not primarily therapeutic, that is, play-related communications, diagnosis and assessments; and second, cognitive-behavioural approaches, since these involve work focusing on the relationship between child and environment and the participation of other adults such as the child's carers.)

1. Therapy is conducted in the context of a therapeutic relationship which allows the expression of the child's feelings.

2. Therapy is based on a common recognition of the function and symbolic meaning of children's play, and the way in which children use play to express their wishes, fantasies, internal conflicts and perceptions of the world.

3. Therapy provides the opportunity for the reworking of trauma, or problematic experiences or events.

4. During therapy, a corrective emotional experience is provided for the child in the context of the child's play.

5. During therapy, the opportunity for the release and ventilation of pent-up or blocked off feelings is offered, and the release of these feelings is seen as therapeutic.

6. Therapy provides the opportunity for the child to develop mastery over feelings, and to a varying extent to develop an awareness of them. Mastery over feelings in turn produces an improvement generally in the child's coping skills.

7. Through therapy, the child's self-esteem, self-confidence, self-image and trust in others is improved.

It is not surprising that within the different forms of play therapy such commonalities of goals and principles should be discernible. Nonetheless, it is necessary, especially in a context which seeks to introduce one particular form of play therapy, to remain aware of the considerable differences which do remain between them. In particular, there seems a philosophic difference between other therapies and non-directive therapy, in that the latter sees the child directing his own activities and the therapist as a facilitator of therapy rather

Table 1. A typology of child psychotherapies.

Degree of therapist directiveness		Approach with child	Focus of sessions	Role of therapist
High	1	Cognitive-behavioural	Making programmes	Design programmes with child
	2	Play related communication	Particular recent event in child's life	Structure session
	3	Structured/focused play therapy	Child's feelings, motives and preoccupations	Structure session
	4	Release therapy	Child's feelings, esp. in relation to trauma	Encourage child to recreate event/ ventilate emotions
	5	Abreactive therapy	Child's feelings, esp. in relation to trauma	Encourage expression of emotional conflict
	6	Psychoanalytic therapy	Symbolism in child's play + dreams/ unconscious material	Uncovering hidden feelings, interpret
Low	7	Non-directive play therapy	Child's feelings, motives and preoccupations	Reflective listening

of events. It may therefore be helpful to think of the therapeutic
῾ong a continuum reflecting the degree of therapist structure and
with those geared to diagnosis and assessment at one end, through
ds of focused play described by Redgrave or Oaklander, through
noanalytic therapy to non-directive therapy at the other. This acknowledges the different degree of therapist control of the interview, whch in turn
may reflect either the purpose of the encounter or the method being used.

S E C T I O N   T W O

NON-DIRECTIVE PLAY THERAPY

HISTORICAL PERSPECTIVE

The non-directive approach to play therapy was developed most fully by
Axline in two books (1946; 1987) and a series of shorter articles and
contributions to edited works on play therapy; the books have continued to
receive a world-wide readership nearly a half-century after they were written.
Although others writing in the same period (notably Allen, 1942; Dorfman,
1976; Moustakas, 1953) also describe this approach, Axline is widely regarded
and cited as its chief exponent. Her first book is devoted entirely to a case study
of play therapy undertaken with a six-year-old boy, Dibs. As an account of the
therapeutic relationship, and an illustration of the way in which an individual
can through play achieve the resolution of and mastery over inner conflicts it
has clearly inspired many readers. In her second book she develops eight
principles of practice for the non-directive play therapist, and links these to a
discussion of the therapeutic process which includes numerous practical
examples of how to deal with common problems in therapy – for example,
the child who is reluctant to leave his mother in the waiting-room; the child
who wants to take toys home; aggressive behaviour; and so on.

It is clear from the regularity with which her work is cited (Dockar-Drysdale,
1970; Wolff, 1986; Clayden, 1986; Mearns and Thorne, 1990; Marvasti, 1989,
to name but a few) that Axline's work continues to be influential in the practice
of play therapy, and that her ideas are seen as forming a distinctive approach
to its practice. Wolff, for example, reviewing the development of child
psychotherapy, selects this as one of three theoretical models in her discussion.
Marvasti (1989) cites this as one of five distinctive approaches to play therapy:
both reviewers, while acknowledging the Rogerian framework in which it is
set, ascribe its development as a form of play therapy entirely to Axline, basing
their accounts on her eight principles, and making no reference to formulations
or developments of other practitioners.

Many writers, too, even when they do not themselves adopt a non-directive approach, acknowledge the relevance of Axline's thinking to their own work. Winnicott, for example, in discussing the 'intensely real' experience of play for the child, comments:

Also, this observation helps us to understand how it is that psychotherapy of a deep-going kind may be done without interpretative work. A good example of this is the work of Axline (1947) of New York ... I appreciate Axline's work in a special way because it joins up with the point that I make in reporting what I call 'therapeutic consultations' that the significant moment is that at which **the child surprises himself or herself**. It is not the moment of my clever interpretations that is significant. (1988: 59)

What is also apparent from a review of the play therapy literature, however, is that although widely read and frequently quoted, Axline's model has failed to develop into a school of thought, tested, modified and with its own training programmes. Where her approach has been adopted, it has tended to be in a somewhat ad hoc, piecemeal way, and to be written up in a manner which is descriptive rather than analytical, and eschews much theoretical exploration. Neusner, for example, describes her approach as essentially non-directive, and her case excerpts support this description: however, the following passage suggests that at times she may incorporate an interpretive approach into her work; and the phrase 'rather passively' suggests an approach which is not consistent with a Rogerian view of the therapist activity of reflection; rather it seems an apparent misunderstanding of it:

The technique I used with Peter could be loosely described as the Virginia Axline type of non-directive play therapy – it was Peter's responsibility to choose activities for each session, and I usually rather passively reflected back to Peter his own play and verbal material (interpretations I made have usually met with stiff resistance as Peter refused to hear what I was saying). (1981: 26)

It may be unfair to criticize this study for its lack of critical analysis or exposition, since it may be argued that such descriptive accounts of practice form a recognizable genre, and do not aspire to theoretical sophistication. We quote it, however, by way of demonstrating the fact that Axline's model, where it has been followed, has been adopted in what may at best be described as an idiosyncratic manner, and one which suggests little attempt to develop a consistent formulated approach to intervention.

Although this is, as we suggest in chapter 1, not untypical of the British approach to practice, it is by no means always the case that practice in this country has developed in this piece-meal, somewhat atheoretical manner. The British school of object-relations theory, for example, first propounded by Fairbairn (1954) and developed by Dicks (1967) among others, has informed the work of the Institute of Marital Studies, and its original formulations have been extended and adapted in for example, marital work and psychotherapy (for example, Mattinson and Sinclair, 1979). The behaviourists, by tradition readier to develop and examine their practice within a theoretical framework, and the family therapists, have also examined and modified their practice with some theoretical rigour (Wilson and James, 1991).

Moreover, even if a certain pragmatism could be said to be typical of British eclecticism, the same cannot be said to be true of North American practice, which traditionally has followed stricter models. Why then has the non-directive approach, so widely quoted, not developed a fuller and more rigorous methodology?

The publication of Axline's work in the late forties, closely followed by Rogers' major work on client-centred (non-directive) psychotherapy (1976) which included a chapter on play therapy, clearly created widespread interest, and the ensuing years were followed by a flurry of articles in the professional journals (Bixler, 1949; Moustakas and Schalock, 1955). Since this period of activity, however, very little of note appears to have been written, so that the majority of articles selected by Schaefer (1976) for a compilation of basic writings on play therapy date from this period.

There are, we suggest, a number of reasons which may explain this. First, the approach appears to have spawned a number of what must frankly be described as rather cranky accounts which make uneasy reading and may have brought the method into disrepute. The case quoted in Axline's article, for example, first published in 1955 and included in Schaefer's volume (1976), would to a sceptical reader appear to border on the reckless:

"Now you've given me a knife and I'll cut your wrists." He suddenly reached out, grabbed the therapist's hand and placed the open blade against the vein. "Now what are you going to do?" he demanded.

"It seems to me that is my question," the therapist replied. "You're the one with the knife. What are you going to do?"

"You wonder what?" John asked.

"I certainly do," the therapist said. (Schaefer, 1976: 217)

Second, although Axline's exposition of her eight principles of play therapy, and subsequent discussion of the enactment of these in practice is clear and rigorous enough, the view of the development of personality and the place of play in the therapeutic process on which they are based is incompletely realized. As Wolff, a psychoanalyst herself, comments: "the exposition of her theories of personality, of its development, and of childhood psychopathology are frankly anti-Freudian and are also unclear ..." and she criticizes Axline's writing for being "entirely unself-critical and at times quixotic". (1986: 227–228)

Furthermore, the links with Rogerian psychotherapy, although discernible throughout, are incompletely explored, and the function of play in the therapeutic process and its relationship to mental and emotional development is barely analysed:

Play therapy is based upon the fact that play is the child's natural medium of self-expression. It is an opportunity which is given to the child to 'play out' his feelings and problems just as, in certain types of adult therapy, an individual 'talks out' his difficulties. (1987: 9)

As we shall demonstrate in the next chapter, the place of play in child development and its function therapeutically is a good deal more complex than this suggests and our discussion will highlight why non-directive play therapy can be powerful and effective without interpretation. Rogers himself was aware of these complexities and touches on them briefly in a discussion of what he terms unsolved issues:

Is the crucial element in the counsellor's attitude his complete willingness for the client to express any attitude? Is permissiveness thus the most significant factor? In counselling this scarcely seems to be an adequate explanation, yet in play therapy there often appears to be some basis for this formulation. The therapist may at times be quite unsuccessful in achieving the child's internal frame of reference, since the symbolic expression may be so complex or unique that the therapist is at a loss to understand. Yet therapy moves forward, largely, it would seem, on the basis of permissiveness, since acceptance can hardly be complete unless the counsellor is first able to understand.

He adds in a footnote:

Since writing the above, a different explanation has been pointed out to the author. It is quite possible that the child assumes that the therapist perceives the situation as he does. The child, much more than the adult, assumes that everyone shares with him the same perceptual reality. Therefore when there is permissiveness and acceptance, this is experienced by the child as under-standing and acceptance, since he takes it for granted that the therapist perceives as he does.

If this description is accurate, then the situation in play therapy differs in no essential way from the description of the relationship which has been given throughout the chapter. (1976: 49–50)

Axline deliberately eschewed an attempt to embed her work in a more fully realized framework, feeling that an atheoretical approach was demanded in order that the child should not be proscribed, and as something of a reaction against the prescriptiveness of the Freudians and the behaviourists. This may, nonetheless, have contributed to the failure of the approach to develop a coherent following.

Third, the principles of Rogerian psychotherapy on which non-directive play therapy is based do seem themselves to have been vulnerable to misinterpreta-tion and frequently to have been imprecisely practised. As Mearns and Thorne point out:

Rogers became somewhat exasperated with those ill-informed critics who took pleasure in depicting him and his associates as passive nodders wedded to a policy of inactivity (1990: 1)

and go on to state their own disquiet at

the recent proliferation of counselling practitioners, both in America and Britain, who seem to believe that by sticking the label person-centred on themselves they have licence to follow the most bizarre promptings of their own intuition or to create a veritable smörgasbord of therapeutic approaches which smack of eclecticism at its most irresponsible. (1990: 2)

Why this situation should have developed in relation to Rogerian psychotherapy must again be a matter for speculation, since those who have trained in and practise it would argue that as a method it demands as rigorous a discipline as any other form of psychotherapy.

We suggest, however, that from its first inception the language and terminology of the approach lent themselves to misinterpretation. In particular, the use of the term 'non-directive' to describe the central essential reflective style of therapist response has been taken to mean that the therapist did very little but mirror, or parrot, the statements of the client. Neusner's small aside, "rather passively", is we would guess, not untypical of the way that the activity of reflection was misinterpreted: reflection which involves an accurate empathic response, and helps the client to recognize and experience more fully his or her deeper and hitherto unrecognized and unacknowledged feelings involves an active and precise use of language and mind on the part of the therapist. It could never therefore be described as 'passive'.

Second, the use of the word non-directive has been frequently criticized for suggesting that the therapist offered, or thought she was offering, the client a completely free rein: whereas again it is quite clear from any reading of Rogers that the therapeutic session **is** directed, that certain activities (for example, a conversational exchange or 'chat' between therapist and client) are discouraged, and that the therapist helps the client to focus on certain feelings and behaviours to the exclusion of others. In other words, the term non-directive is used to describe one essential part of the process, the encouragement to the client to identify and bring to the session what he or she wishes; and to try and distinguish this style from other approaches where the therapist may direct the client to the subject-matter, and, through interpretive comment, to a particular understanding of its meaning. It is not an attempt to encapsulate the whole orientation.

Third, the ideas embodied in person-centred, non-directive counselling appear to have been taken to mean that no boundaries were set, either in the therapeutic relationship or on the behaviour sanctioned. Thus, for example, Marvasti, in an otherwise accurate and certainly neutral exposition of non-directive play therapy, comments: "In this modality of therapy, an extension of Rogerian psychotherapy, there is total permissiveness." (1989: 19)

In fact, the working out of the appropriate limits in play within the therapeutic session is, as we shall discuss in a later chapter, an important feature of work with many children. While we would guess that Marvasti would recognize this, it seems likely that the notion of total permissiveness has been misunderstood, and contributed to the kinds of bizarre practices referred to by Mearns and Thorne.

A further flaw in Rogerian psychotherapy has been its failure to insist on rigorous training for those practising it. The requirement in other psychodynamic approaches, particularly Freudian or Jungian psychotherapists, that the practitioners themselves undergo some form of training analysis has at the very least ensured that psychotherapists within these frameworks have been trained and supervised in the work they are doing, and that, however much ultimately they modify or adapt their approach to suit their personal style, they do so from a clear understanding of the theoretical base of their work. No such control has been exercised in respect of Rogerian psychotherapy. It seems likely that the emphasis on therapy as a shared activity, on the client's ability to solve his or her own problems and the need to deinvest the therapist of the power of the expert has also led to a denial of the skill involved and a hesitation about the need to insist on proper training.

Since non-directive play therapy has its roots in Rogerian psychotherapy, it seems likely that the rather loose way in which the latter has developed and been practised has in its turn affected the development of this mode, and has led to a similar lack of rigour in the way it is practised; an absence of proper training and validation; and a lack of a body of evaluative research which would support its practice and enable it to modify and grow as a result of the evaluation of different aspects of its methodology in the way that other psychotherapies have done.

NON-DIRECTIVE THERAPY/PERSON-CENTRED THERAPY: PRINCIPLES AND PRACTICE

We shall in this section explore briefly the main tenets of Rogerian psychotherapy, consider how these are developed in Axline's basic principles of play therapy, and then consider in more detail how these may be enacted in practice. (The reader is referred to Rogers (1951) and Truax and Carkhuff (1967) for a fuller account and discussion of person-centred counselling.)

In most fields of human activity, divisions into categories or schools of thought are for the most part heuristic, that is to say, they involve the grouping together of things which are more or less alike, and the separation of these from things which are rather less like them, for the purpose of convenience or study. However, it is likely that any such categorization will of necessity cut across similarities between the categories, and suggest a greater difference than may in fact exist. Thus for example, a discussion of the Pre-Raphaelites as a school of painting may emphasize common characteristics of these painters (brilliant colours, realistic representation of the natural world) at the expense of commonalities which they share with painters in their recent past. In the same way, Rogerian psychotherapy, although having certain distinctive characteristics, has also much in common with other psychotherapeutic orientations.

In a discussion of the relationship between non-directive play therapy and other psychotherapeutic work with children, Dorfman makes this general point, demonstrating in particular the similarities between Rogerian therapy and the Rankian orientation, with its emphasis on the relationship between client and therapist, and concluding that the principles of client-centred therapy owe much to the older therapies:

From the Freudians have been retained the concepts of the meaningfulness of apparently unmotivated behaviour, of permissiveness and catharsis, of repression, and of play as being the natural language of the child. From the Rankians have come the relatively a-historical approach, the lessening of the authoritative position of the therapist, the emphasis on response to expressed feelings rather than to a particular content, and the permitting of the child to use the hour as he chooses. (Dorfman, 1976: 237)

The central tenet of Rogerian psychotherapy, as we stated earlier, is that individuals have within themselves a basic drive towards health and better functioning, and that they possess the ability to solve their problems satisfactorily if offered the opportunity and the right climate in which to do so. Given this drive and inherent ability, Rogers saw the therapist's role as being the creation of the right conditions in which this 'self-actualization' can take place. He believed these to be characterized by three elements, or 'core conditions' as they are frequently described in the literature, and much of his writing explores how they are worked out in practice. These characteristics of the therapist may be described as:

Genuineness and authenticity: that is, the capacity to be real, to be themselves as distinct from adopting a role or defensive posture with the client.

Non-possessive warmth: an attitude of caring and engaged and friendly concern, without becoming overly emotionally involved or offering help for self-serving reasons. (This is similar to Rogers's unconditional positive regard, with the amendment of 'non-possessive' to draw attention to the need for a measure of detachment on the part of the counsellor.)

Accurate empathy: the ability to feel with those who are seeking help, and articulate these feelings, so that the client feels understood, and is helped in turn to a greater understanding of these feelings.

As we suggest in the opening paragraphs of this section, it should not be held that Rogerian psychotherapists have a patent on the use of these core conditions: indeed, as Truax and Carkhuff (1967) among others have demonstrated, although the research evidence suggests that therapists who possessed or had learned these three core traits or attitudes produced beneficial effects beyond those observed in equivalent control groups, the theoretical approach adopted by these therapists is relatively insignificant.

For our purposes therefore, in addition to these core conditions which arguably pertain in any effective relationship (although they receive most emphasis in Rogerian psychotherapy) the essential characteristics of non-directive counselling are that the therapist is responsive to what the client is saying, and reflects back to the client his or her understanding of what the client is experiencing. Through this process of accurate reflection the client is helped to greater recognition of feelings, and the beginnings of mastery over them.

The reflection is in a strict sense non-interpretive, in that it remains in the present, uses on the whole the material that the client has used and avoids what has been described as the 'now and then' kind of interpretation, that is, one that links current material to past events. Thus Axline defines reflection as the "mirroring of feeling and affect"; as such it is communicated by the therapist within the metaphor used by the client (unlike for example in psychoanalysis where what the client says or does may be interpreted and the metaphor transposed into what it appears, to the therapist , to be representing.) In working with adult clients the 'content' is likely to be verbal: with children the metaphor is frequently, although not necessarily, play.

Axline, in developing non-directive play therapy, incorporates these Rogerian principles into eight guidelines for practice. In her writings she develops them largely through accounts of working with the child's play, but they are in essence a reformulation of Rogerian principles, involving as they do an emphasis on the development of a trusting accepting relationship between practitioner and client; an acceptance that the client chooses the direction the session is to go in; reflection rather than interpretation; non-intrusiveness and a respect for the client's defences; and the setting of appropriate, therapeutic boundaries to the relationship:

1. The therapist must develop a warm, friendly relationship with the child, in which good rapport is established as soon as possible.
2. The therapist accepts the child exactly as he or she is.
3. The therapist establishes a feeling of permissiveness in the relationship so that the child feels free to express feelings completely.
4. The therapist is alert to recognize the feelings the child is expressing and reflects those feelings back in such a manner that the child gains insight into his or her behaviour.
5. The therapist maintains a deep respect for the child's ability to solve problems if given the opportunity. The responsibility to make choices and institute change is the child's.
6. The therapist does not attempt to direct the child's actions or conversation in any manner. The child leads the way; the therapist follows.
7. The therapist does not attempt to hurry the therapy along. It is a gradual process, recognized as such by the therapist.
8. The therapist establishes only those limitations necessary to anchor the therapy to the world of reality and to make the child aware of his or her responsibility in the relationship. (Axline, 1987: 73–74)

Axline also makes the point (1987: 89) that the process of non-directive therapy is so interwoven that each principle overlaps and is interdependent on the others. Thus a belief in the power of the individual to resolve problems also carries with it the acceptance of that person essentially as he is, the readiness to allow him the choice as to whether, how, when and at what pace to work on issues which may be troubling him, and a willingness to respect his decision about this. This acceptance, giving the client the freedom and right to choose and respecting the decision, does not however mean that the practitioner is merely a passive observer in the sessions. Far from it: creating the climate in which the client is enabled to work things out and helping him or her to discover the capacity to do so, involves the active participation and intense involvement of the practitioner throughout the session. We have found it helpful to think of these principles as embodied in certain practice skills, which we consider here briefly under different headings.

Structuring

Acceptance, the establishment of a trusting therapeutic relationship, means that the worker must demonstrate respect and value of the client through the way in which the sessions are established, namely:

1. A clear agreement with the child of where, when, for how long and how often the therapy will take place.
2. The use of a private room, which is free from interruptions by telephone calls or from other people, and where the child will not feel overlooked by people outside.
3. The establishment of a clear time boundary (usually of an hour), so that the child's rights to use the time as he or she wishes are respected.
4. Consistency in the setting out of the room, and the play materials which are available.

Listening and attending

Accepting the child, going at the child's pace, reflecting feelings and helping the child to greater awareness of feelings all require an intense concentration on the part of the therapist on what the child is saying or not saying, or doing, and on the minutiae of non-verbal signs.

1. It is important to allow the child space to share what he wants to communicate – that is, the conventional rules for talking to someone do not apply. The therapist is not carrying on a conversation, and every pause does not need to be filled with speech, or every gap filled with a question which might provide interesting information. Social conversation is two people alternately waiting to communicate their point of view to one another. Therapy is not conversation; it is client-centred listening.
2. The personal and specific significance in what the child says or does must be looked for (which does not necessarily mean that it is commented on immediately).
3. The non-verbal clues which help the practitioner understand how the child feels about what she is saying or doing must be sought.

4. The feelings about what is being said must be listened to as well as to the words.

5. Any incongruity should be noticed between words and body language (for example, the laughter while describing some painful event) which may indicate tension or suppression of feeling concerning the material which is being enacted or described.

6. The therapist should listen to what is being said in the here and now – trying to link it (as the session is continuing) to past events can distract and break both the child's and the therapist's concentration. (Of course in reviewing the session afterwards, the therapist's drawing on her knowledge of the child's past history to enable her to make sense of and reflect more accurately the child's communication in the light of previous understandings of the child, is essential.)

7. The therapist should also listen to her own feelings while the child is talking or playing. These act as a barometer, indicating what is going on. It is therefore important for the therapist to know what feelings are out of the ordinary for her, so that she can be clear about what 'belongs' to the child and are feelings which are being transmitted from the other person (see below).

8. the therapist should constantly question whether or not she understands how the client feels. Above all it is important to concentrate and try to 'hear' what is being said and felt, maintaining a listening 'openness' to anything the child may choose to say or express.

Accurate empathy: communicating and reflecting

Central to this method of working is the belief that the child or individual has within himself the capacity to resolve his own problems, and that this involves the recognition, experiencing and sometimes the release of emotions which have been denied, concealed or avoided by some mechanism of defence. Part of the means of coming to this recognition and release is through the experience of being recognized, accepted and understood; but part of the process requires that the therapist enables the child to reach a greater awareness of what he or she is feeling. This process involves the ability to hear and correctly identify the emotions which the child is experiencing, and the ability to communicate this understanding in such a way that the child not only feels accepted and understood, but is helped to recognize feelings of which he may have been barely conscious, or have been perplexed and confused by before – as one child put it "you've helped me feel connected up".

1. In responding therefore to what the individual is saying or doing, the therapist tries to de-emphasize the surface content, and respond to the deeper content of what is being communicated. This may help the child to a greater awareness of what he is feeling; it may communicate the therapist's understanding of what the child is experiencing, and give permission for further exploration of these feelings; and may help the child to feel less isolated and cut off by what he is experiencing.

For example, in an early session, a ten-year-old talked almost non-stop about a football game he had been watching, describing parts of it again and again. The therapist reflected her feeling that the child seemed almost frightened about what he would feel if he stopped talking, thus reflecting what she felt was the feeling behind what he was saying. The boy seemed to respond to this, in that he stopped talking, moved closer to the worker and began to draw with increasing intensity.

2. Another means of helping the child get in touch with feelings is by the therapist following the child's lead, rather than attempting to direct the child to what should be talked about, or taking control actively. For example, it is a mistake to attempt to direct the child to where he left off the previous week. Experiencing indecision, hesitating, remembering and so on may be a necessary part of getting in touch with feelings. Giving the child time and space to do this is a vital part too of demonstrating acceptance and respect, and a means whereby the child may experience the exercise of autonomy and control.

3. Having attended and tried to understand what the child is feeling, the therapist should reflect this understanding back in such a manner that the child gains awareness and understanding of feelings and behaviour.

We explore this skill of accurate reflection more fully in a later chapter. Aspects of it are considered briefly here:

(a) Communicate your knowledge of what the child is feeling or experiencing, and root your comments in specific observations of the child's behaviour. By doing this, you help the child's self-awareness to extend to a deeper stratum of hidden meanings and motives, and also help to clarify for the child how he relates to you and to others.

(b) Emotions are predominantly expressed through body language – as you become sensitive to how a feeling is communicated, share this with the child. Again, this helps the child's self-awareness and by locating the understanding in observed behaviour stops the reflection from seeming like a magical insight, the source of which is inexplicable. Of course, one cannot always make the connection between intuition and observation rapidly enough – acknowledgement that you as the therapist experience something, but do not know why, is appropriate.

(c) The reflection of feeling needs to be tentative, without judgement. It should be tentative rather than dogmatic in tone because the comment is made for the child to make use of, pick up or leave as desired – its rightness or wrongness is only important insofar as it helps the child move on – not to prove something for the therapist.

(d) The reflection needs to be made briefly, in language the child can understand, but without repeating the exact words, parrot fashion, which can be irritating.

4. The reflective comment should be free from blame or criticism. Even if the criticism is not overt, it can sometimes be conveyed through facial expression

and tone of voice, and will make the child feel defensive. We realize of course that it is not always as simple as this – we would want to distinguish for example between criticism, which implies a judgement, and feeling uncomfortable, which may be an accurate reflection of the fact that the child has transgressed the therapist's personal and appropriate boundary of self, and should be shared with the child. We return to this later.

5. Avoid asking a lot of questions, particularly in order to obtain further information and facts. Often there is a mass of information on file about the child, but the child's behaviour is not changed as a result and the problem still remains. Asking questions, particularly why, may convey to the child that the therapist does not understand why he is behaving in a particular way. It may leave the child anxious, because he is being called upon to explain behaviour which is perplexing to him also and his feelings of helplessness are ignored. Asking questions shifts the child away from immediate awareness of feelings and behaviour to a demand for an intellectual/verbal explanation about them. The here-and-now experience is lost in attempts to give an explanation of it.

6. A distinction, however, should be made between information or explanation seeking questions and those which are exploratory and are posed in order to help the child identify feelings – for example, a therapist, sensing that she was too close to the child and that the child was feeling threatened by this, asked him if he wanted her to move a little further away, at which the child nodded and as the therapist moved away began to play more freely.

7. Avoid giving advice. Non-directive therapy is not problem-solving, and often the nature of the child's problem is not receptive to advice. Giving advice moreover maintains the therapist in a position of authority, rather than empowering the child to resolve the problem.

8. Avoid interpretation. An analytic approach to the child maintains the therapist as an authority who stands outside the child's problem, and interprets rather than empathizes. Winnicott comments:

If only we can wait, the patient arrives at understanding creativity and with immense joy, and I now enjoy this joy more than I used to enjoy the sense of being clever ... The principle is that it is the patient and only the patient who has the answers. (1988: 102)

9. Resist the sometimes powerful temptation to reassure or comfort. It is often difficult not to step in and offer comfort, but to do so interrupts the child's process of experiencing, understanding and mastering feelings, and again sets the worker in a position of authority, even if a loving authority. Often too the impulse to console comes from the therapist's own need to move away from the experience of painful emotions, rather than being truly child-centred and rooted in the wish to help the child towards mastery.

10. Avoid generalizing about the child's experience, again sometimes from the impulse to reassure or offer advice – for example, "All young people feel this

way". This diminishes the uniqueness of the child's experience, and the focus on the experience gets lost.

Congruence, authenticity and the recognition of personal feelings

In any counselling activity, it is vital that the person offering help has what has been described as the quality of transparency – a willingness to be seen for what one is, without being self-preoccupied or concerned with one's own image. A sense of personal security and self awareness enables the therapist to be open and receptive to the feelings and experiences of others, and frees the person seeking help from the need to take the anxieties and sensitivities of the counsellor into consideration when deciding what it is safe to say or do, and how he may express himself. Moreover if the person offering help is unaware of how he or she reacts to certain situations or feelings, it becomes difficult to disentangle in the therapeutic encounter what feelings belong where. And it is difficult to offer consistency and genuineness if experiences which the client recounts produce unlooked for responses in the therapist.

It sometimes seems difficult to stress the need for personal qualities of warmth, congruence and receptiveness without sounding as if only a saint is capable of doing the work. Of course this is not so: it seems indeed likely that anyone who is able to respond sensitively to the pain of others must derive this at least in part from an awareness and mastery of personal difficulties themselves. What does however seem essential is that anyone involved in counselling should ensure that they avail themselves of supervision which will increase their self awareness and cultivate an attitude of mind which is self-critical.

From what has been said earlier about listening and communication, it will be clear that the feelings which the therapist experiences with the child are an essential part of understanding and reflecting back. Within the session therefore, it is important to use these feelings.

1. If the therapist has been emotionally engaged with the child, it is probable that the feelings experienced will be directly related to what the child is feeling. It is therefore important for the therapist to be aware of:

- feelings which are out of the ordinary.
- feelings that are persistent, for example a pervasive sense of sadness.
- a change of mood which occurs when with the child, for example, a therapist in one session found himself feeling unaccountably and suddenly angry.
- intuitive feelings, such as the sense of anxiety which one may be unable to attribute to anything identifiable.

2. By acknowledging these feelings and sharing them with the child, where appropriate and at the child's readiness

(a) the emphasis on the verbal content of the interaction is lessened or removed.
(b) the child is helped to be more aware of his or her own feelings.

(c) an openness about what is being felt as well as said is demonstrated.

(d) the unspoken interaction between practitioner and child is clarified.

(e) a focus is maintained on the here-and-now.

3. In developing an awareness of how to respond to the child, the therapist needs to be alert to the possibility that experiences outside the session may be having an impact on what she is feeling within it. Usually it is possible to set this aside, sometimes by taking a break for a few minutes before the session. Occasionally, however, these feelings can be so intrusive that some explanation has to be offered to the child, who will be quick to pick up that the therapist is abstracted or anxious.

4. It is important to avoid comparing personal experiences with the child, as this shifts the focus away from him, breaking his flow of self-awareness. The therapist's responses should focus on the uniqueness of the child's experiences, rather than on similarities to other people's or to the therapist's own experiences.

5. For the same reason, the therapist should not share personal details or personal information, since this again shifts the focus away from the child.

6. Sometimes in the course of therapy, the child may seek information, either about the therapist, or about the experiences of other children. In responding to this, it is important constantly to keep in mind whether the sharing of information or experiences is for the benefit of the child, or in order to fulfil the therapist's own needs. The therapist should above all keep in mind the child's feelings behind the questions.

7. Sometimes a child may act in a way which makes the therapist feel uncomfortable. For example, often children who have been abused have no boundaries between themselves and adults or other children and do not know what appropriate physical contact is. It is important for the therapist to reflect back to the child, uncritically, her own feelings, for example, "that doesn't feel comfortable to me", because only through a genuine setting of boundaries can the child learn to identify his own, and distinguish between different physical and emotional expression of feelings. Obviously, the therapist must herself be clear as to what is appropriate.

8. Nonetheless, it is important to consider too the impact that the therapist may have on the child when sharing particular feelings. Sometimes the child's sexualized approaches, or the experiences being recounted, may produce a confusing range of emotions, some of them in turn sexual. It is usually inappropriate to share these sexual stirrings with the child. Equally, there are occasions (for example, in the experience with a very obese girl described in chapter 3) when it feels too potentially wounding to share one's responses. The issue of whether and how to respond in situations where a range of uncomfortable emotions are aroused in the therapist is complex, however, and we shall return to it in a later chapter.

We have in the last section of this chapter highlighted the main principles and practice skills involved in non-directive play therapy. In the next chapter we consider the theoretical foundations of this approach, and the framework within which these principles and skills should be understood.

— 2 —

Symbolic Play: Its Role in Mental Development and in Play Therapy

In order to discuss the importance of play to a child and its role in therapy, we intend to set both child's play and child therapy within a broader framework of mental development. By showing the theoretical foundations on which we are basing our non-directive play therapy, we shall demonstrate that this form of therapy derives its effectiveness and rationale from basic principles of mental development.

These principles were not developed by Axline or by the other non-directive child therapists (see chapter 1) largely because of the historical and theoretical context in which non-directive play therapy emerged; child therapy and child development usually had divergent audiences and interests. Currently, however, therapeutic writing acknowledges child development theory and research and their applicability to individual cases (see, for example, Wolff, 1989; Barker, 1988; Stern, 1985). Piagetian theory is often viewed as compatible with a therapeutic approach; emphasis is given to the relationship between the way a child thinks and his emotional responses to events. Areas within child development, such as attachment theory and research on emotional understanding, also highlight current rapprochement.

Our aim in this chapter, then, is to show that non-directive play therapy can be set broadly within a Piagetian framework and within current knowledge of mental development.[1] By demonstrating that non-directive play therapy is a reasoned and theoretically based therapeutic approach to children, its effectiveness in the treatment of children can be more readily understood.

The first part of the chapter will present general principles of mental functioning, introducing the concepts of adaptation and symbolic play as highly assimilative adaptive activity by a child. We shall then discuss the child's mental organization, conceptualized as being based on personal and objective schemas.

Conceptually, these schemas are separated into affective, cognitive and motor components, but all are experientially unified. We then make some general assumptions about consciousness and the relation of schemas to a child's conscious awareness, including the role of coping (defence) mechanisms in conscious activity.

Our discussion then turns to symbolic activity, and the way mental imagery and language are related to non-directive play therapy. We conclude the first part of the chapter by arguing that play materials are used as external symbolizations of thought in a child's play and by discussing the varied functions of play in a child's mental life and their relation to non-directive play therapy.

The second part of the chapter is intended to clarify for the reader how non-directive play therapy makes use of the features of mental development we present in the first part; these features, we shall argue, are inherent in all children's normal development. We shall discuss first the way symbolic play activities are utilized within non-directive play therapy. Second, we shall discuss ways in which past experiences are reintegrated into current functioning by the child. Finally, we shall illustrate the manner in which a non-directive play therapist uses therapeutic techniques such as structured exercises and role playing to enable the child to make therapeutic progress.

ADAPTATION, ASSIMILATION AND SYMBOLIC PLAY

Following Piaget and other organismic theorists, all of a child's activity during his development is assumed to further his adaptation to his environment (see Figure 1 on pp. 38–39 for a schematic illustration of the discussion that follows). Adaptation always consists of two functions, accommodation and assimilation. The child continuously takes in or assimilates his surrounding environment to his own ongoing activity; he also adjusts himself, or accommodates his activity, to his environment. A child from birth onwards is assumed to assimilate actively every external person and object he interacts with, as well as his internal activities, into his past experiences. This active internalization of experience, or assimilation, is seen as the most basic activity, and one that is more elemental than accommodation.

Symbolic play activity, on which non-directive play therapy is based, is a highly assimilative activity for a child (Piaget, 1962). This feature of play helps account for the ease with which children engage in symbolic play both under everyday conditions and during therapy. While this feature of symbolic play is not expressly stated by Axline (1947), she does refer to the adaptive nature of the child's activity. Axline assumes the child in non-directive play therapy is constantly interacting with his environment, and therefore constantly changing and learning.

An example of an assimilative process in concrete play terms is the interaction of a child with a play object, say a policeman's hat. The child can choose to assimilate the hat to his play activity by pretending that he is carrying a bucket, that a monster fell on his head, or that it is a hill for a car to climb over, thereby engaging in highly assimilative activity by disregarding most of the hat's characteristics. The hat is being used symbolically in play, then. But the child must still accommodate to the object's characteristics to a certain extent by taking the shape of the hat or its function into account when he uses it.

As the above example demonstrates, adaptation is potentially very flexible because systematic and varied use of symbols can be exploited by the child. Unlike intelligent action, which is largely under voluntary control (see Piaget, 1967), certain mental activities are largely self-regulating ones. Dreaming, day-dreaming in adults, and symbolic play in children, all assimilate events symbolically, largely without any conscious attempt to accommodate with the environment. In symbolic play a child freely assimilates his experiences to personal (mental) schemas, with few constraints imposed by the environment. For this reason from symbolic play a child derives a feeling of freedom as well as "the joy of self-expression" (Erikson, 1977: 42), simply because external constraints can be largely ignored (Axline, 1947).

ORGANIZATION BASED ON SCHEMAS

Along with adaptation the second major principle guiding a child's development is organization (Piaget, 1952). Adaptation and organization are inseparable: adaptation is the externalization of the child's underlying internal organization. The child's activity is never an isolated act in itself; it is always related in a systematic way to his other similar acts. Separate parts of this system, according to Piaget, are organized into structures called 'schemas'. Based on schemas developed from past experience, a child is predisposed to act similarly in the present. But it is assumed that these schemas are not completely determined by the past – instead they are 'mobile frames' applied to different situations.

The organization of the schemas is constantly changing because, as well as assimilating new events to past experiences, schemas must also accommodate to the specific features of the current situation. This accommodation means that the organization of the schemas themselves must change. The schemas undergo internal differentiation; there is increased discrimination of objects and situations in which the schemas apply. In addition, schemas continually form more complex and interconnected relationships with other schemas during development.

Stern, in his exploration of the way an infant experiences himself and others, argues that an infant does have a sense of self, and "emergent self", which is based upon the infant's "... subjective experiences of various organizations in formation ..." (1985: 60). This view seems similar to Piaget's, where internal organization and external adaptation are inseparable. They are different ways of conceptualizing the same phenomena. Stern states that the organizational processes involved in forming an infant's sense of 'self' and 'other' are complementary to the view of infant experience which asumes that an infant first perceives separate featural elements of persons. This featural view of infancy uses theoretical constructs such as:

... assimilation, accommodation, identifying invariants and associational learning. The emergence of a sense of self is therefore described more in terms of discoveries about the relations between previously known disparate experiences than in terms of the process itself. (1985: 61)

When the organizational process itself is the focus, Piaget assumes that experienced events are organized internally by a child into schemas which are constantly changing through assimilation and accommodation. This provides a richer theoretical basis for Axline's statement that a child's developmental process is a cumulative, integrative one (Axline, 1976). It also clarifies and broadens our understanding of therapeutic progress. For a child who makes therapeutic progress, the process of therapy seems to produce a change of personality organization and structure, as we shall illustrate in the next chapter. Rogers also states that "the essential outcome (of therapy) is a more broadly based structure of self, an inclusion of a greater proportion of experience as part of self". (1951: 195)

Therapeutic progress, then, can be viewed as involving schemas increasingly assimilating new events to past experiences. Because of the increased assimilation begun in therapy, the underlying organization of the schemas themselves change and they change their connections with other schemas. Further, underlying and underpinning this process of change "... are the forward-moving forces of life itself ... and because of this deeper force the individual in therapy tends to move towards reorganisation rather than towards disintegration." (Rogers, 1951: 195).

PERSONAL AND OBJECTIVE SCHEMAS: AFFECTIVE, COGNITIVE AND MOTOR COMPONENTS

Schemas can be broadly divided into personal and objective schemas; that is, schemas connected with persons and schemas involving objects. Each personal or objective schema has an affective, a cognitive and a motor component to it. It is assumed, then, that affect,[2] cognition and motor attitudes are inseparable experientially, and components of all three are involved in each mental state. While every schema has affective, cognitive and motor components, the degree of each component varies. Objective schemas are usually highly cognitive and personal schemas are mainly affective.[3] Piaget sometimes refers to schemas which are predominantly affective as 'affective schemas'; similarly, predominantly cognitive ones are called 'cognitive schemas', and schemas which are primarily motor predispositions are known as 'motor schemas'.

There are many gradations of schemas. For example, Wellman notes that some cognitive attitudes "possess a definite affective or emotional coloration ... Examples are approval and boredom. These sorts of attitudes (it's boring that the game was cancelled) can be termed cognitive emotions because the affective component requires much prerequisite cognition." (1990: 114)

Piaget assumes that affective schemas do not usually achieve as much mobility and generalizability as cognitive schemas do, and remain more completely assimilative in nature. The extent of affective schemas' mobility and generalizability has recently been explored by Harris (1989). His research into children's development of emotional understanding, that is, the cognitive component of personal schemas, seems to show that children at early ages engage in complex expression of their emotions (for example, young children shifting between affection and anger in their behaviour towards family members) without conscious recognition that this ambivalence exists in themselves. In normal development a child seems gradually to realize on a conscious level (say, by about age ten) that he can experience mixed feelings and does not insist that positive and negative emotions are mutually exclusive, as he did when younger. Harris concludes that this developmental process can best be described as "a genuine case of the child turning round on his or her own schemata, and gaining new insight as a result". (Harris, 1989: 125)

Harris also gives evidence that under certain emotionally difficult circumstances, say hospitalization, less mobility and generality of the cognitive component of affective schemas occurs. Young children, and older children with emotional problems, seem to express ambivalent (and other complex) emotions without having the ability to be consciously aware of both emotions together. That is,

the child engages in a thorough analysis **at some automatic or semi-conscious level** [our emphasis] that leads to the overt expression of ambivalence in behaviour. (Harris, 1989: 125)

With emotionally troubled children, then, affective schema do not seem to be very mobile. This has important implications for therapeutic work with children experiencing difficulties in their emotional development.

Complex and conflicting emotions will be expressed, but cannot be consciously analysed and verbalized by the child (Harter, 1977). Harter found that conflicting emotions expressed by troubled children she worked with included smart–dumb, love–hate, good–bad, happy–sad, and others. She spontaneously discovered while working with a six-year-old girl that drawing two polarized emotions made them concrete and manageable for the child. Drawing, modelling, role playing, verbalizing, etc. all seem to help troubled children in middle childhood more easily gain cognitive insight simultaneously into both poles of these emotional continua. (We shall discuss this technique in more detail in the second part of this chapter.) However, in general it seems that all children throughout middle childhood are only gradually achieving cognitive insight into complex emotions. As we state above, the level at which therapeutic insight occurs in young children (and, indeed, in older children and adults at times) will be largely at a 'semi-conscious' or experiential level, rather than a cognitive level; often the symbols will have private meaning rather than social meaning.

CONSCIOUSNESS AND MENTAL DEVELOPMENT

In play therapy, then, young children gain largely experiential insight into their emotions, and older children develop both experiential and cognitive insight. In order to understand the way this insight occurs, it is important to consider the role of consciousness in mental development. The mind seems to be constantly active, regardless of whether or not the person is consciously aware of his own mental activity. In order to become consciously aware of mental activity, assimilations must simultaneously activate corresponding accommodations to form a mental equilibrium. Assimilation by itself, whether it is affective or cognitive, is largely outside of awareness. It is the end-results of mental activity, as translated into symbols, that become conscious, rather than the on-going thought processes themselves. Unlike psychoanalytic theorists, unconscious mental activity is **not** assumed to congeal in a special region of the mind and it is **not** confined to affective activity. Every mental process varies in its degree of, and possibility for conscious awareness (Piaget, 1962; Walls, 1972).

As we have already discussed, personal schemas are highly affective and predominantly assimilative in character. Therefore, besides the immediate symbol that the person can be consciously aware of, there may be more remote meanings of which he is unaware, which he has assimilated to the symbol. Some thoughts, for instance, may seem 'pregnant with meaning' to the person. An example which seems to demonstrate this kind of activation of a personal schema is given by Freud:

If a few bars of music are played and someone comments that it is from Mozart's **Figaro** (as happens in **Don Giovanni**), a number of recollections are roused in me all at once, none of which can enter my consciousness singly at the first moment. The key phrase serves as a port of entry through which the whole network is put in a state of excitation. (1900: 535)

In this case a stimulus activated a personal schema which could not find full symbolic expression immediately. Several potential symbolic representations could be worked through thought by thought; several thoughts may merge and condense into one image; perhaps the mind becomes occupied with other symbolic representations of ongoing events and the schema is left undeveloped; or perhaps the thought is threatening to the person and the thought is either blocked, denied or distorted.

Because thoughts of troubled children in play therapy are particularly likely during their previous development to have been activated and then blocked, denied or distorted, it is especially important to examine types of mental coping strategies commonly employed by children under stress.

COPING MECHANISMS AND CONSCIOUS AWARENESS

A dramatic illustration of the way highly self-threatening experiences are blocked or distorted by the child using mental coping strategies is contained in a study by Pynoos and Eth (1984) of children who have been witnesses to homicide. Some of the mental coping strategies these children used were: repression, in which the child attempted to block all spontaneous thought to avoid traumatic content; fixation to the trauma, in which the child repeatedly gave an incomplete, journalistic retelling of the traumatic event; displacement, in which the child transferred feelings about the trauma itself to fearful feelings about his own future harm; denial-in-fantasy, in which the child imagines a positive outcome rather than the traumatic one; and identification, in which the child identifies himself with the police or one of his parents.

Other coping strategies such as detachment, in which the child becomes withdrawn, numb or mute about the traumatic event or displays greatly heightened anxious attachment (especially younger children) are noted. Motor coping strategies, such as repetitive, unsatisfying traumatic play, sometimes involving other children, and, more dangerously, re-enactment of the traumatic event in real life are also described.

Another coping mechanism, not discussed in this study, but which is highly relevant to children subjected to sexual abuse, and discussed at greater length in chapter 6, is dissociation, an extreme form of denial. In sexual abuse, where the child himself is directly involved in the experience, the child may split his motor actions away from his feelings and mental activity in order to cope with his recurring abuse.

Unlike adults, who more often have post-traumatic amnesia, young children who are witnesses are more likely to express their anxiety directly in the immediate aftermath of a trauma, rather than to use this cognitive defence (coping) mechanism (Pynoos and Eth, 1986).

However, when the child is directly involved in recurring abuse, amnesia does seem to occur. It appears likely that cognitive coping mechanisms gradually develop in children, in keeping with their general level of mental development and are more basic and transparent than in adults, as are lies (Ekman, 1989) and emotional understanding (Harris, 1989). Children use coping mechanisms to deal with abnormal anxieties, as illustrated above, and to deal with normal, everyday anxieties. By middle childhood coping mechanisms have developed to deal more effectively with anxiety and guilt (Barker, 1988; Wolff, 1989); by adolescence coping strategies largely resemble adult ones (Pynoos and Eth, 1986). (The reader is referred to the general literature for a more detailed discussion on coping mechanisms.)

The development of coping mechanisms has immediate relevance to non-directive play therapy. The therapist, rather than dealing directly with the child's coping mechanisms, instead has the child freely assimilate his mental activity in a non-threatening environment. The therapist attempts to help the child make conscious and give symbolic representation to thoughts which are largely outside of conscious awareness. That is,

One of the most characteristic and perhaps one of the most important changes in therapy is the bringing into awareness of experiences of which heretofore the child has not been conscious. (Rogers, 1951: 147)

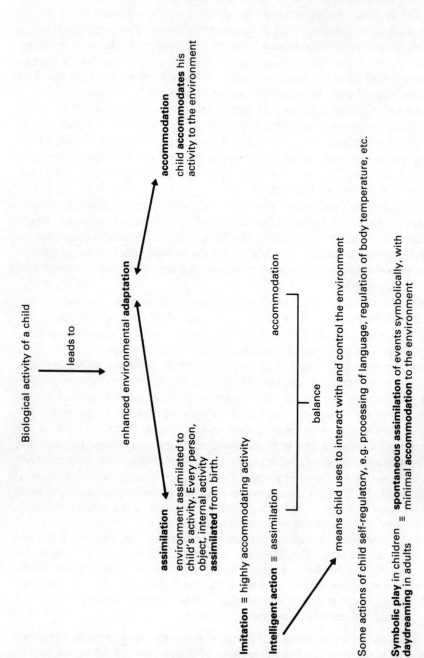

Biological activity of a child

leads to

enhanced environmental **adaptation**

assimilation
environment assimilated to child's activity. Every person, object, internal activity **assimilated** from birth.

accommodation
child **accommodates** his activity to the environment

Imitation ≡ highly accommodating activity

Intelligent action ≡ assimilation

balance

accommodation

means child uses to interact with and control the environment

Some actions of child self-regulatory, e.g. processing of language, regulation of body temperature, etc.

Symbolic play in children **daydreaming** in adults

≡ **spontaneous assimilation** of events symbolically, with **minimal accommodation** to the environment

≡ free assimilation of experience to personal (mental) schemas; environmental constraints largely ignored

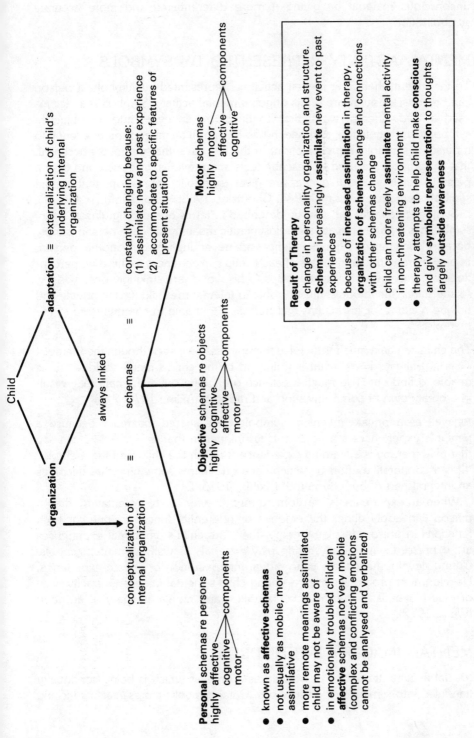

Figure 1 The relationship of play therapy to mental development.

The therapist, then, tries to enable the troubled child to deal with previously unconscious material by giving it more differentiated and more accurate symbolization.

MENTAL ACTIVITY REPRESENTED BY SYMBOLS

To the extent, then, that mental activity is represented by symbols, a person can be consciously aware of his ongoing mental activity. Symbolic capacity is used in two different ways: first, to transform an event into an objective symbolic representation; and, second, to transform an inner or outer event into a personal symbolic representation. In the first case, the symbol is referential; that is, symbols are used to describe facts about events. In the second case a person's feelings about events are given symbolic expression; that is, the symbol is emotive (Cassirer, 1944; Chomsky, 1966; Rado, 1969).

Symbolic capacity can also be described in terms of meaningfulness. Every symbol has a purely private and idiosyncratic meaning for each person, simply because each person's life experiences are never duplicated in another person. In play therapy the uniqueness of each child's experiences, of his own perceptions of himself and his relationships to his world, are strikingly observed. As Axline states, the therapist must be able to tolerate the child having private and unique reasons for his actions that he may be unable to communicate to the therapist:

The child can gain much from (play therapy sessions) even though the therapist does not always know what is going on in the child's inner world – and is unable to find out. Too much insistence on finding out everything may result in a breakdown of communication and rapport. (Axline 1976: 215)

As well as a private meaning, symbols have shared meanings because a person's experiences are never totally unique. In that sense, Axline can say that play therapy is a learning experience for both the child **and** the therapist. "It is a cooperative effort by which each one learns something that becomes an integral part of both of them." (Axline, 1976: 215)

When an experience is transformed into its symbolic representation, then a person can apply either the emotive or referential function alone, or both functions in unison. In play therapy, then, the child's emotional experiences are expressed symbolically, using play materials as well as mental symbols. During development there is a gradual internalization of private experience. Development progresses from a young child's mental images and active use of play materials to the inner verbalization and mental imagery of an adult (Walls, 1972).

MENTAL IMAGERY IN CHILDREN

Mental activity, then, can be viewed as a process which is being continually translated into symbolic representations. Outer symbolic representations include play, language, and later, drawing, music, role playing and poetry, for example. Two different types of inner symbolic activity are mental imagery and inner speech. Mental imagery, to be discussed first, includes reproductive imagery, anticipatory imagery and memory imagery. Reproductive and anticipatory imagery combine constructions from current schemas; memory imagery is directly related to past experiences in a person's life (Piaget and Inhelder, 1969).

Mental imagery, according to Piaget, is a means of mental representation which is independent of language and objective concepts. That is, "... symbols such as images, memories, symbolic objects, etc. are inherent in the individual mechanisms of thought". (1962: 70) Mental imagery, in Piaget's view, depends on and develops from a child's 'deferred imitation' at about two years and not from his language development.[4] By forming mental images of events and persons, a child can imitate a model in the model's absence. The child can retain events in memory for longer time periods than when the events had only sensory motor representation, as at earlier stages of development. Also the child is able to engage in pretend or symbolic play, mentally to evoke events which are outside his immediate perception. (Piaget, 1962)

An example Piaget gives which illustrates that mental imagery is dependent upon imitation yet independent of language, is becoming consciously aware of imitating someone, but being unable to figure out who it is. Piaget noticed that he was smiling differently and realized that he had formed a mental image based on the earlier experience of noticing a stranger on a train, who smiled that particular way as he read. (Piaget, 1962)

Many psychologists note that mental imagery in children is more vivid than in adults (Werner, 1948; Schachtel, 1959; Richardson, 1969, for example). Richardson makes the distinction between a common adult form of remembering, in which memory images are used only as 'signposts' to past experiences, called 'abstract verbal memory', and the usual kind of childhood remembering in which mental imagery is used almost exclusively, called 'concrete image memory'. Richardson demonstrates the difference between these two forms of remembering in this way: in abstract verbal remembering we "retrieve the fact that I went sunbathing yesterday and that I saw Bill on the beach ..." In concrete image remembering we "retrieve in quasi-sensory-affective form a re-experience of the sights, sounds, smells, tastes, pressures and temperatures that were involved in the original experience". (1969: 141)

It is the use of concrete image remembering that explains the ability of young children, who are unable to articulate complex emotions and thoughts in language, to remember and recognize past personal events accurately. A dramatic example of a young child's recall using mental images is a three-year-old girl's accurate recall of her experiences and assailant when she was kidnapped and sexually assaulted (Jones and Krugman, 1986).[5] She clearly had a fuller recollection of her experience than she could express in language. (See also the example of David in chapter 7, section 3.)

Another feature of concrete image remembering is the role mental imagery plays in children's thoughts, not just when subject to traumatic events themselves, as above, but also when they are witnesses to such events. In the study mentioned earlier by Pynoos and Eth (1984) children who are witnesses to homicide, especially a homicide involving one or both parents, have vivid and highly disturbing images of these events. As Richardson described above, these images are a 'reliving' of the event, with the power of highly personal (the child's 'worst moment') and sensual evocations; they are not inner verbalizations or abstractions. Pynoos and Eth demonstrate that it is by giving these personal memory images overt symbolic representation with the help of a therapist – through talking about them, playing through the scene or drawing them – that the child is able to gain some mastery over these mental images.

In play therapy, then, especially with younger, pre-school children, mental imagery will predominate. Representation of thoughts by mental images seems to be the mode preferred by the child even after he can use language to communicate with others.

While verbal and conceptual thought is collective thought and therefore inadequate to express individual experience, mental imagery (as a mode of representation), on the contrary, is created by the child for his own use, and the egocentricism of the signifier is then exactly suited to the nature of what is signified. (Piaget, 1962: 155)

FEATURES OF THINKING IN MENTAL IMAGES

We shall now examine the special features of thinking in mental images. The most basic feature seems to be that, in contrast to verbal thinking, images are immediately experienced by the person's mind and the person is immersed in the images he is experiencing mentally. In symbolic play and day dreaming, the hypothetical nature, or the 'if-ness' of the experience, is maintained, while in dreaming the person's immersion is almost complete.

Mental images are adapted, manipulated and changed through two underlying mechanisms common to all mental functioning: the process of synthesis and the process of differentiation (Werner, 1948; Cassirer, 1944; 1955). These two mechanisms operate at their most advanced level in abstract thinking and at their most rudimentary when thinking in mental images. The most rudimentary form of differentiation is displacement, while the most rudimentary form of synthesis is condensation (Piaget, 1962; Gill, 1967).[6] In condensation, diverse meanings are unified into one image. Different situations and images are assimilated to one another as the contents of different personal, affective schemas are expressed and a new image created. For example, a child who is playing that his imaginary space ship is stopping for petrol is condensing two different meanings into one image. Displacement, on the other hand, means that the image shifts in meaning. The child's image, that is, tends "to fade and blur from one meaning and form into the other ..." (Werner, 1948: 156) The meaning that is altered is based upon personal salience, rather than objective criteria. An example of this kind of displacement is seen in young children's story-telling. Having heard a story from another young child and being asked to repeat it, children do not relate the story using an objective sequencing of events from beginning to end. Instead, the events are sequence-based upon personal, affective criteria (Piaget, 1948).

It is predominantly through mental images, then, that the young child will alter his personal, affective schemas in play therapy. Mental images, both current and memory images, will be condensed and displaced. These images will be incorporated into the child's play experience with the therapist and result in emotional insight into his experience. It is the use of mental images, then, that explains the child's ability to express even complex emotions appropriately. These are the symbols operating on the "automatic or semiconscious level" referred to earlier (Harris, 1989) without the child having the ability to be consciously aware of his emotional responses. The therapist, then, must attempt to follow these mental images and play out (as well as verbalize) with the child the affective, personal content of these schemas. It is evident, then, that an essential feature of therapeutic work with young children is that the therapist is able to appreciate the nature of the young child's thought patterns. As Axline states:

The child may not always seem rational in his communication from an adult's point of view and yet, from the child's frame of reference, he is communicating real down-to-earth feeling. A therapist who is too literal-minded and who cannot tolerate a child's flight into fantasy without ordering it into adult meaningfulness might well be lost at times. Few adults have the flexibility and creative spontaneity of a child. (1976: 623)

By adapting to the child's thought patterns the therapist can help the child in this non-threatening environment to re-experience and re-order his perceptions and gain emotional insight:

Therapy is basically the experiencing of the inadequacies of old ways of perceiving, the experiencing of new and more adequate perceptions and the recognition of significant relationships between perceptions. (Rogers, 1951: 222–223)

LANGUAGE AND MENTAL ACTIVITY IN CHILDREN

Another essential skill of the therapist in play therapy, as we stated earlier, is verbally to reflect feelings which the child is expressing during the session back to the child himself. How, then, do the therapist's and the child's verbalizations influence the therapeutic process? We shall now discuss this second type of symbolic representation of mental activity, language.

Bruner et al. (1966) and Piaget (1962) assume that imagery is the significant means for cognitive processing in early childhood and is gradually replaced during development by linguistically based cognitive operations. Unlike mental imagery, which is largely personal and private, language is based upon social convention. Collectively shared experiences, thoughts and objects are represented by arbitrarily agreed sounds and sound patterns. Children learn that objects have names and these names are organized in a systematic (grammatical) way to give meaningful utterances. By its nature, then, language – and later 'inner speech' – is more amenable to abstraction and generalization than imagery is. The relationship between the thing signified and the signifier (the word or image) is imposed by social convention for language, but in imagery the relationship between signifier and signified is a spontaneous one which is directly experienced by the person (Cassirer, 1955; Piaget, 1962).

When a child learns a particular language, certain relationships and experiences he has will be emphasized and others ignored; language, unlike imagery, will not mirror his personal experiences (Whorf, 1956; Sapir, 1958). In general, then, a child will be discouraged from using language idiosyncratically as he develops and will be encouraged to follow conventional usage.

Language, like imitation, becomes internalized during a child's development. This interiorization of language occurs much later than 'deferred imitation' or mental imagery. By about seven years children seem to be able to represent thoughts systematically to themselves and to control their actions using inner speech (Vygotsky, 1962). Inner speech begins effectively to regulate both internal mental activity and overt behaviour.

In normal development, as communication becomes more complex and a child's mental processes also increase their complexity, the child learns to distinguish between thoughts which can be expressed openly and those thoughts which should be expressed mentally and privately, even though potentially communicable. In emotionally troubled children this process has often been disrupted. In creating a permissive environment, the therapist also must create a private environment without interruptions and interference from the outside world. In doing so, when the therapist gains the child's trust, the child is then able to use the therapeutic situation as one in which private thoughts and actions, previously unable to be expressed, are permissible without criticism or ridicule. The child can then come to realize that even though some thoughts and actions may be prohibited by his environment, they may still be expressed symbolically, either through play and other overt formal symbolic representations, or on a private, mental level of mental imagery and inner speech.

Certain types of environmental experiences seem to nurture the child's ability to use mental imagery simultaneously with language (or 'inner speech') to represent his personal experiences. A child seems to learn this capacity in an environment in which parents are verbally expressive, discussing plans and shared memories with the child. It also seems to be fostered by the child's own storytelling and talking about his own hopes and memories (Singer, 1966). In non-directive play therapy the permissive, child-oriented environment which is created also nurtures the child's use of mental imagery in conjunction with the language from the therapist, and in conjunction with his own outer and/or inner speech.

MENTAL IMAGERY, LANGUAGE AND PLAY THERAPY

In play therapy we are attempting to heighten a child's insight and self-understanding by fostering conditions in which a child can learn simultaneously to use mental imagery and language (and/or 'inner speech') to represent his personal experiences. In that way both the cognitive and the affective components of personal schemas will come to be integrated at the child's current developmental level.

We also assume that through symbolic actions using toys and play activities a child's motor schemas will be re-integrated into his cognitive and affective schemas. (Specific examples are discussed more fully in chapter 6.) For this reason, it is essential that the therapist verbalize the child's thoughts and feelings about his personal schemas, rather than simply participating in the child's play, although at times, as mentioned earlier, the therapist will have an incomplete notion of the mental images and experiences that the child is attempting to integrate.[7] In order to reflect thoughts and feelings effectively back to the child, the therapist's verbalizations must be an accurate reflection of the thought processes of the child, even though perhaps rudimentary and incomplete. The degree of verbalization will be partly dependent upon the age of the child. With a largely non-verbal child, say a three-year-old neglected child who has the spoken language of an eighteen-month-old at the 'telegraphic' speech stage, the child is able to benefit from play therapy largely by re-experiencing and reintegrating his mental images with the help of the therapist. The therapist, by creating a permissive environment and responding to the non-verbal cues of the child, will create a feeling of empathy and non-possessive warmth.[8] Reflections of feelings through language will be necessarily rudimentary, often focusing on key words such as 'happy', 'sad', 'naughty', 'big' as the child expresses these feelings in play and in his relationship to the therapist.

It is also necessary to be aware that a young child's production of speech may lag behind his ability to comprehend speech (Flavell, 1985).[9] The child may be able to understand words for the feeling states he represents in his mental images and in his play when used by the therapist even though he does not use them himself. The therapist needs to be aware that her speech to the child will, ideally, be slightly beyond the child's ability to produce speech, but within his listening competence. In effect, the therapeutic environment is potentially an ideal language learning environment for the child, especially in relation to emotive language. Indeed, research findings in language acquisition demonstrate that a young child who has access to much semantically relevant speech, that is to adult speech which is directly related to the child's activities, interests, intentions and vocabulary, seems to have his language development accelerated (Snow, 1986). Another side-effect of non-directive play therapy seems to be that it can accelerate the child's cognitive functioning because the child is reintegrating his personal schemas, both their affective **and** their cognitive and motor components

At the same time as affective reintegration, more purely cognitive activities such as using language to communicate feelings and thoughts, or learning about using numbers or the ordering of objects into classes seem to be freed to develop. We have noted that often substantial gains in cognitive learning occur as mental images and language are reordered at a more appropriate developmental level. This effect, as others we noted, needs to be explored more systematically by further research.

For a verbally and cognitively more advanced child, the therapist needs to change her level of verbalization to the child accordingly.[10] This ability to speak at the child's verbal level of development, while it may seem daunting on the face of it, is naturally present in many parent–child communications and, arguably has a built-in, biological basis which an adult would then be able to exploit consciously in a therapeutic situation (Lenneberg, 1967; Snow, 1986). The spoken language of a four- or-five-year-old is often more advanced, yet his thought processes have many of the nonconserving features described by Piaget which are important to take into account. For example, a young child unable to conserve on a mental level, takes one feature of an object into consideration when making a judgement and then sequentially notes another feature. This type of thought is applied to personal schemas using mental images as well. In therapy the child 'thinks about' as well as plays out his past and current experiences. The child's mental images may, for instance, be one in which the child is hurt by the parent and another one, perhaps sequential in his actual experience, in which the parent gently strokes the spot where he was originally hurt. A young child, using the therapist in the role of the child, and himself as the parent, might play out the mental image of being hurt by pretending to slap the therapist across the cheek with his hand. As the therapist reacts appropriately by pretending to be hurt and frightened, the child might then enact his other mental image of the parent lovingly stroking the child's cheek, with the therapist responding that the child (parent) wants to be gentle now, that it feels good now where the cheek had been hurt.

Developmentally, the child will be unable to understand the complex motivations of the adult who hit him and then stroked him where he had been hurt. His emotional understanding and thoughts about the event will remain on a sequential level of understanding (see Harris, 1989). However, substantial gains in both affective and cognitive control will be gained. First, and most basically, he will now be able to think consciously about and recall these events. Second, he will have reordered his mental images of his experiences by enacting them in a permissive environment using play materials symbolically. Third, by taking the role of the parent, as well as seeing his own role enacted by the therapist, he will move beyond the egocentricity he experienced in the original event. And, fourth, with the therapist's verbalizations, he will hear, and be able potentially to use himself, words to describe the emotions he previously only felt and reacted to. In all the above ways, both cognition and language will be advanced, and his emotional understanding and mastery of these personal experiences will be increased.

PLAY MATERIALS AS EXTERNAL SYMBOLIZATIONS OF THOUGHT

Let us address more specifically now the external means which a child uses to give symbolic representation to his personal experiences, his play. As well as using mental symbols and language to represent experiences, as discussed above, a child needs to make these experiences more concrete for himself by using toy materials and engaging in play activities. A child, because of his limited mental and language abilities, needs materials and activities to symbolize externally his thoughts and feelings: "Just as language makes subtle and complicated thought possible, perhaps toys do the same for play." (Newson and Newson, 1979: 12) Among the needs of children that toys fulfil are the needs "to explore, to invent, to create, to test out their skills, to show off, to stretch their physical limits, to fantasize, to role-play and to act protectively to something less powerful than themselves". (Newson and Newson, 1979: 69)

In non-directive play therapy, as our earlier discussion of play materials indicates, a range of materials is selected to enhance and fulfil these different needs. Because of the non-directive nature of this kind of therapy, a child can experiment with different materials and activities at different points in therapy and thereby choose the means that are most suitable for himself symbolically to represent personal experiences. Some children may find sand the right medium to express their hostility, by burying a figure in the sand, while other children may crash cars together or throw balls at a target. Or one child may use all these different means of expression in one play sequence.

FUNCTIONS OF PLAY IN A CHILD'S MENTAL LIFE

Turning from toys and materials to the play activities themselves, many theories of childhood play have been offered: 'traumatic' theories of play view play as serving the function of repeating symbolically experiences not sufficiently mastered in the past, thus gaining active mastery over them; developmental theories of play stress play's functional purpose in promoting learning and exercising new abilities, thereby preparing for the future; and cathartic theories discuss play as a means of releasing surplus energy, which engenders a sense of well-being in the child (Huizinga, 1949; Piaget, 1962; Erikson, 1977).

All of these functions are to some degree present in all children's play. In fact, as argued earlier, play can be seen as a self-regulating activity, whose function is to assimilate events freely, largely without constraints by the environment. In non-directive play therapy as well, an artificial and enhanced play environment is created in which play serves the role of mastery, learning and release from painful emotional experiences and feelings.

A further essential of all play, however, is that play can be satisfying, and even joyful, because it contains "the uniqueness of the child's own personality ... Potentially each child's play is the perfect expression of (himself) as a developing individual". (Newson and Newson, 1979:12) In the permissive and private

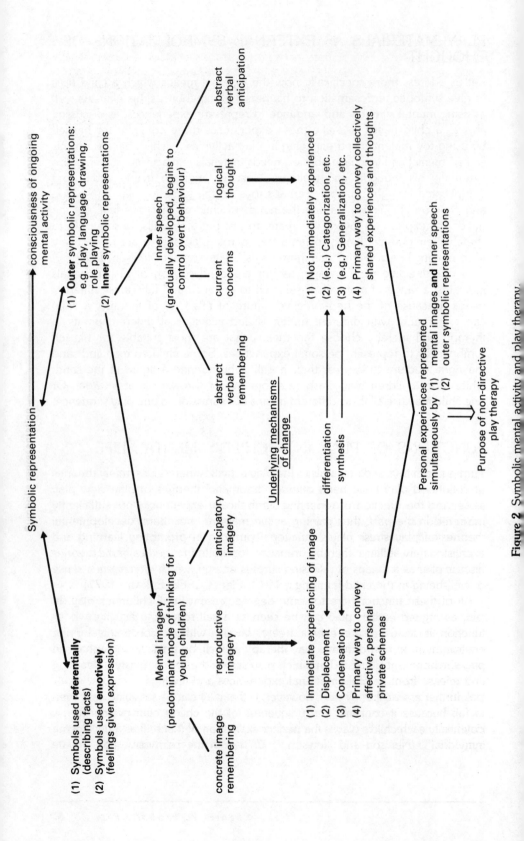

Figure 2 Symbolic mental activity and play therapy.

environment which has been created therapeutically, a troubled child can play out the uniquely affective, personal contents of his affective schemas which, unlike emotionally healthy children, he has been unable to do otherwise. Many children at different stages in non-directive play therapy react, like Axline's Dibs (1946), with deep pleasure, wonder and satisfaction in finding that they can play with what they want in the way they want. They seem to be recognizing consciously, perhaps for the first time, that they are finding acceptable expression for their unique personal feelings.

A further characteristic of play on which the effectiveness of non-directive play therapy depends is that "play offers a stimulating environment for both intellectual and emotional creativity". (Newson and Newson, 1979: 12) This is because play depends upon either the absence of agreed rules, such as private idiosyncratic symbolic play, or the implicit acceptance of rules as social conventions developed from mutual consent in social games and rituals. That is, "play is not a behaviour **per se**, or one particular type of activity among others. It is determined by a certain orientation of the behaviour ..." (Piaget, 1962: 147) Because of this orientation "wherever playfulness prevails, there is always a surprising element, surpassing mere repetition or habituation". (Erikson, 1977: 17) Newson and Newson (1979) also recognize that play is supremely flexible because even though a child may have rituals or established and familiar patterns of behaviour, it is

because these are (his) own rituals, (he) has the right to jettison them at any moment and to move off in entirely new directions at will. It is this supreme flexibility which makes play the ideal setting or jumping-off point for creative thinking and imaginative invention. (Newson and Newson, 1979:12)

This characteristic of play is maximized in non-directive play therapy. By the therapist creating a permissive environment and trying to respond as a child directs, rather than the therapist giving structure to the play, the child can change his play at will. This stance even applies for more structured games devised by older children. A school-age child (say seven years onwards) is cognitively more mature than a younger child and potentially has mental imagery, inner speech and language available to represent his emotional experiences. When an older child introduces a game, say soccer, the child would be the one to introduce and direct the game, interpreting the rules to the therapist, which can change according to the child's needs. By having flexibility of rules, the child can then play out personal emotional experiences in his game with the therapist, involving such complicated emotional relationships as fairness, cheating, luck, punishment, co-operation, elation, pride, satisfaction and anger. Both the personal and the social meanings for the child can be united concretely in this one symbol.

We assume that symbolic play evolves into a variety of both social and personal activities from the symbolic play of earlier childhood. Symbolic play, as above, develops into social games; it also evolves into spontaneous daydreaming in older children and adults (Walls, 1972), as well as into formal symbolic expressions such as music, art and drama. In working with older children, media such as drawing and sculpting can be aids to representing concretely complex feelings. Role playing activities also can become increasingly elaborate, with the child enacting dramas with different characters. We shall examine some of these activities in more detail in the second part of this chapter.

Therapists often attempt to help a child symbolize experiences by introducing concrete forms as aids to emotional understanding (Oaklander, 1978). These structured exercises introduced by the therapist, such as "the empty chair", are concrete representations used primarily to advance the child's cognitive understanding of emotional experiences. As such, they have a useful, but limited role. Sometimes a child's increased cognitive understanding can be a route for altering his personal, affective schemas, just as sometimes a motor activity, such as soccer illustrated above, is a route. But at other times role playing or water play may be a more effective and potent route. In non-directive play therapy, with the child discovering and exploring his own routes with the aid of the therapist, the individual child can design his own self-chosen therapy, rather than having it imposed on him by the therapist.

By playing spontaneously in non-directive play therapy, then, the child can play with both his thoughts and his feelings, which results in "a kind of imaginative free-wheeling". (Newson and Newson, 1979: 12) Play which began as aimless and unfocused can become clarified and crystallized, leading in specific directions, and then turn back into being aimless again, either within the session, or for the next play session.

To summarize, through symbolic play troubled children spontaneously work through emotions experienced in frightening and confusing situations. The therapist's role is to enable the child to have the security and self-confidence to express private experiences and to try out different ways of thinking and acting in his play. That is,

The client becomes aware of experiences which have not been previously accepted. He also becomes aware of the fact that he is the perceiver and evaluator of experience, a fact which seems to be very close to the heart of therapy. (Rogers, 1951: 210)

Even more importantly, through playing in non-directive play therapy, the play experiences themselves are transformed into "acts of renewal" by the child (Erikson, 1977). We shall demonstrate more fully in the second part of this chapter how a child's re-enactment of experiences symbolically during non-directive play therapy results in a reworking of his mental schemas and are, for him, "acts of renewal".

SYMBOLIC PLAY

We shall now discuss the way symbolic play activities are utilized within non-directive play therapy.

A child, as we have stated, uses toys to represent his emotions and thoughts symbolically. Puppets, for example, are an especially potent means of representation because puppets are more personal than objects. In a sense, when the child wears the puppet on his hand or arm, the puppet becomes an extension of himself, yet still removed from actually being himself. The child can distance himself from the emotions, thoughts and actions of the puppets, and can, if needed, reject and deny them as his. But puppets can also take on their own life and movements and become 'real' for a child more easily than objects. It is easier with puppets, then, for a child to identify with them and have them take on human characteristics. It is also interesting to note that animals are easier, often, for children to use to convey their emotions, thoughts and actions than toys with human features, such as dolls. Perhaps this is because animals are both further removed from humans, and thus less threatening, as well as being without language, and thus more amenable to embodying emotions through actions.

Sometimes even less animate symbols are used by the child to convey personal meanings. For example Plate 1 shows how a ten-year-old girl expressed a variety of feelings about herself and her need for emotional support. Using a symbol of herself as a rose, she painted herself as one rose among many, explaining that the other roses represented her friends. She conveys her emotional involvement with her father (and his friend) by portraying them also as roses, but towering over her. (Her father was at this time still in prison for sexual offences against her in which his friend had also been implicated.)

This view of symbols highlights a major difference between the psychoanalytic and non-directive therapeutic approach. Non-directive play therapy attempts to respect the child's symbols, rather than interpreting them, and attempts to follow the child's inner experiences through symbolic means if the child chooses to express himself symbolically rather than concretely. Instead of the psychoanalytic relationship with the child of dependency, transference and counter-transference, the non-directive approach attempts to forestall these problems within a therapeutic relationship by letting a child keep the defences (coping mechanisms) and symbols he chooses to use unless he feels able to give them up himself, rather than depending upon the therapist to direct his progress, and to interpret and unmask his symbols and defences.

When a child plays on a symbolic level, characteristics usually emerge in his play and can be used therapeutically. First of all, the child usually identifies himself most with one of the symbols. If the therapist looks for the symbol with the most emotional significance to the child, she will be able to empathize more accurately with the child's emotions and actions. In Helen's case, to be discussed in the next chapter, she used the monkey puppet as herself and her sister seemed to be identified with the elephant puppet. But in other cases the child's emotional identification is not as straightforward. Sometimes a child splits good parts and bad parts of **himself** between puppets. Older children sometimes enact complex puppet shows with many characters. It then becomes more difficult to identify clearly the child's 'alter-ego(s)'. Second, the child's use of symbols, if not taken too literally, allows the therapist to understand what a child thinks and feels more deeply, often, than a child is able to express in any other way. The child, too, can see his emotions, thoughts and actions more objectively, because they are removed from himself – in fact, with puppets, for example, they are truly "at arm's length". (Newson and Newson, 1979)

Another characteristic of a child's symbolic play is that a toy's actions often fulfil an emotive function. Especially in the early stages of working with troubled children, a child will use toys symbolically to represent his personal conflicts in thoughts and emotions. The therapist, by focusing on the toys' actions and commenting on the emotive meaning behind the action, can both get the tone for therapeutic work by conveying obliquely to the child that the sessions will deal with his emotions, at the same time as helping the child to maintain his defences against anxiety. For example, a child might play with a toy train, continually running the train off the track and having it crash upside down. The therapist, while keeping in mind that the train may represent the child himself, will attempt to find the emotional basis for the action, and, depending on the context, may comment on the train being out of control, that the train always goes too fast on the track so that it comes off the track, that the train can't go and needs help when it's upside down, etc.

Often this kind of play sequence is marked by repetitions of one theme, and indeed at times it seems likely that the child has often repeated this sequence himself in solitary play. But the difference now is that the therapist is helping the child to clarify the feelings and thoughts behind his play and the child is showing the therapist, on a symbolic level, where he feels one or more of his difficulties lie. By working on the symbolic sequence together, the child sometimes spontaneously comes to a creative solution to the toys' difficulties. Other times the child seems to recognize consciously what the toys' problems are, repeating some of the therapist's comments to himself or to the therapist. And at other times the child seems to be caught up in his problem, unable to have any emotional distance from it and simply feeling similar feelings with the toys, but in the therapist's presence.

Depending upon the child's reactions during symbolic play sequences, the therapist is able to make some tentative inferences about the child's therapeutic progress on the problem he is representing. It is important for the therapist to realize that while at times she will see creative solutions to symbolic play representing the child's difficulties, at other times the child may, after clarifying his problem symbolically, work on this problem in the intervening time between sessions. If the child seems to be actively – both mentally and emotionally – working on the play sequence, it seems likely that he will continue this therapeutic work between sessions and/or in the next session. (This is one of the reasons why it is important for the therapist to keep to the time limit, as we discuss in chapter 3.) If the child seems unable to work actively on the play sequence with the therapist, he might not yet be ready to deal consciously with the problem. In either case, the non-directive therapist has faith that the child, when he is able to, will find his own unique solutions to his problems. This partially removes the overwhelming burden sometimes felt by therapists (and others in the helping professions) that it is their sole responsibility to 'make things right' for the child.

Another way symbolic play can be used by a child is to represent his feelings about his relationship with the therapist. If he feels angry with the therapist, but feels threatened when he becomes angry with adults, he may represent the therapist with one car and himself with another car and continually crash into the first car. As with other symbolic play, the therapist would convey the thoughts and feelings of the child, using the child's symbols, yet being aware that it is likely that the child is feeling aggressive towards the therapist. By being aware of the problem or individual that the child is representing symbolically, the therapist will be more accurate in her empathy with the child.

It is usually more difficult for the therapist to realize when the child is representing their own relationship symbolically, because of the lack of distance and lack of objectivity which characteristically occurs when a person is herself engaged in a relationship. Especially when the therapist has difficulty accepting certain feelings in herself – say that she feels guilty at being unable to extend the sessions because of work pressure – it is often difficult for her to recognize the child's symbolic representation of their relationship. The child may, for example, try over and over again to build up a high sand castle, but no matter which way he builds it, the sand castle falls down. If this play sequence occurs when therapy sessions are ending, the child is often symbolically representing his feelings of frustration and helplessness over the therapeutic relationship itself ending. Or perhaps his frustration and anger, depending on the quality of the play sequence, is due to the therapist having just had two weeks' holiday. It is necessary for the therapist to realize that, while language clarifies and helps a child consciously deal with emotions and thoughts represented to himself symbolically, and are a crucial part of the therapeutic process, symbols and symbolic play **in themselves** carry meaning.

As we discussed in the first part of this chapter, ongoing mental activity is translated into symbols. It is these symbols, whether formed as mental images, language or action (motor) memories, which are conscious. With personal affective schemas, assimilation of thought is predominant over accommodation and for young children it is largely based on mental images and actions. For younger children language is not used as readily to represent inner experiences. The child is in the process of **developing** the ability to use language to represent shared inner and external experiences.

Language, as we discussed earlier in this chapter, is one of the primary means of sharing experiences, of developing a sense of mutuality and understanding between people, based on the shared meanings of words. As language develops the child's ability to utilize inner speech increases (Vygotsky, 1962) and begins to interact with mental images and outer actions to represent his personal experiences to himself. This process, however, is incomplete during childhood. Even at about nine and ten years of age a child often uses 'props' to play out his private thoughts and fantasies (Singer, 1966) – say by using a small figure and moving its arms while whispering to himself. The actions of toys at each stage in a child's development are used as adjuncts to his thought processes, and help to make concrete these rapidly changing mental images. The therapist, too, is using the same methods the child uses to help make conscious the child's inner experiences. Through directing the child's attention to words which can be used – and shared – to represent his private thoughts, by acknowledging his actions in play as his symbolic representations of inner experiences, and by helping the child to concretize his inner experiences with toys which stand for mental images, the therapist is reinforcing a spontaneous ability that is developing to represent experiences that all children possess. The therapist is also acknowledging that all these modes of representing experiences interact: words can call forth personal experiences (the word 'ice cream', say, would evoke different feelings and memories in each of us); actions have their own power to evoke memories and feelings (say, riding a bike evoking the feeling of being on holiday and being carefree) and a mental image, of, perhaps, a snowy mountaintop, evoking personal feelings of coldness and isolation or of peace and solitude to different people. It is when all of these means of representing personal, affective schemas are used simultaneously or sequentially, as in non-directive play therapy, that symbols become a powerful means of representing and creating personal experiences, and are in themselves significant to the child (and to the therapist).

In playing as well, the child can use a toy to represent powerfully and creatively his personal feelings. For example, a neglected ten-year-old boy who suffered from epileptic seizures, in using a foal leaning against a mare, then falling and struggling to get up to try to lean against the mare again, is experiencing a poignant and powerful personal symbol of his inner experiences. This kind of symbolic play can have varied and remote meanings and experiences attached to it of which both the child and the therapist are not consciously aware, because such play involves relatively permanent affective schemas. These meanings may not find full symbolic expression, and words may not be adequate to describe these experiences, but "Let a person get even a glimpse of the truth, a tiny portion of success, and if this is really incorporated into one's self-system, a change occurs." (Corsini, 1966: 25) The symbolic representation itself, then, has power and can help instigate change.

The symbolic mode of representation is also, of course, seen in the paintings and drawings produced by children in play therapy. Just as some children seem to prefer role playing, discussed later, or using the sand box to work out their conflicts, other children spontaneously paint or draw. As with other forms of action-based symbolic representations, it is important for the therapist to comment verbally on an affective level and to use the symbols provided by the child in his artwork (unlike psychoanalytically oriented therapists, who would attempt to interpret the child's drawings). At other times the therapist needs to be reticent, to withhold her comment because it might break the child's concentration which he needs to produce the painting or drawing or enact other play sequences. In these cases it is often better to let the play action or painting itself produce its emotional effect on the child and briefly comment only on an obvious feature – say the size of the sun and how warm it must feel or how fast the train is going – in order for the therapist to show the child that her attention and support is with him. (For further examples see chapter 7.)

All of these symbolic representations we have discussed can have emotional importance for a child and can give the therapist understanding of the child's progress in therapy as well as of his unique personality style and mode of mental (and concrete) imagery.

REINTEGRATION OF PAST EXPERIENCES

We shall now discuss the means a child uses in non-directive play therapy to reintegrate his past experiences. Every child who makes therapeutic progress seems actively to reintegrate his past experiences into his current level of development. The child re-experiences his past in the therapeutic situation and integrates this past into his current functioning. Sometimes the therapist glimpses the child re-experiencing his past, for instance when a child plays with toys which he recognizes as belonging to his earlier life. But it does not seem to be enough that the child simply plays with younger toys or plays on a less mature level with the toys in the playroom. It seems essential that the child himself recognize that he is doing so.

Some toys and materials, certainly, lend themselves to re-experiencing earlier events and feelings more easily: sand, water, playdough, a baby's bottle, a drum, to name a few. These materials seem to involve physical sensations and actions – the child's whole body – rather than simply being objects that are played with. Some of these toys have been labelled 'hypnotic' toys (Newson and Newson, 1979) because the whole body is caught up in a rhythmic action with the toy. As with daydreaming in adults (see Walls, 1972), rhythmic action using toys or materials is a relaxing experience for a child. Even more, it seems to project the child into a different level of awareness:

It seems to occupy just enough of the attention to free the rest of the child's awareness for creative and imaginative thought. Perhaps it fills up that part of the consciousness which would otherwise be distracted by more demanding stimuli ... children often do a lot of thinking as they swing gently to and fro. (Newson and Newson, 1979: 17)

The child's play with 'hypnotic' toys is somewhat similar to certain adult hypnotic states. In an adult hypnotic state the hypnotist puts the person into a relaxed state in which a different attitude about events and experiences is made possible for the adult (Lee et al., 1976).

It is more, then, than the child simply regressing to a less mature level of functioning. The child by playing with younger toys, is able to re-experience creatively an earlier level of development, at the same time still being aware of his present developmental level. Younger children seem to do this largely through actions, while the therapist verbally recognizes the feelings attached to their actions and acts herself in response to the child's actions and instructions.

A three-year-old boy, James, was referred to play therapy after being removed from home and sent to live with foster parents because of emotional and physical neglect and possible abuse by his mother and stepfather. Negative behaviours he exhibited while still living at home were smearing his bedroom walls and floor with excrement and severe temper tantrums. During his play therapy sessions James played with Fischer-Price little people in the dolls house, several times locking the little boy in the upstairs room and saying, "It's dark in there." The therapist, reflecting his feelings, said, "The boy is frightened ... The boy is all alone in the dark ... The boy doesn't like it." (It is especially important with younger children for the therapist to convey verbalized feelings clearly through her voice tone and facial expressions in order to make the message clearer.)

James, in a following session, discovered that he could instruct the therapist to lift him up so that he could reach and control the light switch by himself. This was an important achievement for him: after his first success, he did a little dance of joy in the middle of the room. In a later session James was able to re-experience his past through actions; he not only seemed to recreate his past, he seemed to integrate it into his current experiences. In a following session James deliberately tried to be naughty by throwing sand around the room, and the therapist reflected these feelings: "You want to be naughty ... You want to make me cross." James was then able to instruct the therapist to lift him up to the light switch, while he held sand tightly in one of his hands. He would then turn the light switch off, hurtle the sand from his hand on to the floor below and then turn the light switch on again. He repeated this sequence twelve times, one after the other, while the therapist carried out the actions he required of her. The therapist made comments, such as: "You can do the light **yourself** now ... You want to make a mess ... You're very cross with the light off." James was able, it seems, to recreate the traumatic feelings he experienced when being punished and locked in his room in the dark, his own anger and smearing while being in the dark, and his ability now to control the light switch while he re-experienced these emotions.

Older children are often more able than younger children to verbalize their remembrances of past experiences for themselves. For example, a ten-year-old girl talked with fondness of a favourite doll she had when she was little, as she undressed one of the dolls in the playroom. This kind of re-experiencing using speech and toys is characteristic of a child in middle and late childhood, who has not yet fully internalized private experiences and seems half-way between daydreaming and playing. An adult may be able spontaneously to verbalize these remembrances during therapy, and thereby integrate them into current emotional functioning, but an older child still seems to need toys as props and cues for his mental activity. And because these feelings are based on private experiences and feelings, perhaps never shared or made conscious before, it is most likely that children will reintegrate past personal feelings and events into current development at later stages rather than early in the therapeutic process. Another common way that older children recreate past experiences is through role playing and puppetry. In both cases the older child is able at times to immerse himself in the actions; the feeling states and events become very real and are re-experienced by him in a new way.

Sometimes in play therapy a child relives experiences in a deeper, more personal, way. Ekstein, for example, writes: "(During) a later phase of therapy ... the child threw the ball repeatedly for the therapist to retrieve and in ecstacy clapped his hands, saying 'dada' **like a small baby**". (our emphasis) (Ekstein, 1966: 108). Children may also induce a trance state in themselves by sucking, as does Helen, whom we describe in chapter 4. In Helen's case, and in Jeffrey's case in the later chapter on sexual abuse, and in the above examples, the child seems to recreate his past experiences and integrate these emotionally healthier re-enactments into his current functioning.

THE ROLE OF STRUCTURED EXERCISES IN NON-DIRECTIVE PLAY THERAPY

As we discuss in more detail in chapter 5, the child in middle childhood uses concrete objects and concrete experiences to arrive at correct solutions to problems. This feature of children's thinking in middle childhood helps explain why structured exercises are advocated by some child therapists, notably Oaklander (1978), but see also Harter (1977). Structured exercises such as 'the empty chair' or 'three wishes' have evolved out of therapists' attempts to explain complex and difficult emotions to children in middle childhood. Children at this stage in their mental development are gradually achieving cognitive insight into complex emotions. Before middle childhood structured exercises are largely unproductive because young children have not developed cognitive schemas necessary for analysing and achieving cognitive insight into difficult emotions; they use mental symbols and motor schemas to achieve experiential insight.

However, once a child can consciously work on a cognitive level, concrete exercises can be an effective and preferred mode of therapeutic resolution to problems for some children. And certainly, given the slow evolution of cognitive insight into complex emotions for even emotionally untroubled children, the use of concrete experiences and objects to arrive at emotional solutions to problems can be effective in adolescence and even into adulthood. Similarly to role-playing, clay modelling, puppetry and other play activities described in this book, structured exercises also have a place in the repertoire of the non-directive play therapist. The therapist ideally needs a working knowledge of many different therapeutic skills in order to help the child clarify his emotional conflicts and work towards creative solutions. By responding to the spontaneous and sometimes tentative explorations of the child in an assured way, the therapist can help the child develop his preferred method(s) of working on his problems. Harter illustrates a therapist's effective use of a concrete representation to advance emotional understanding:

... later in the treatment ... the scene was (yet) another command performance during which I was being chastised by the teacher (that is, the child in the teacher's role) for not paying attention to the lesson and for doing poorly on my math. I finally donned a look of extreme frustration and raised my hand ... "Teacher, teacher, I just **can't** concentrate on my math, I can't think, there is something that's bothering me, and I want to tell you how I am feeling." ... I persisted ... Finally I asked if I could come up to the blackboard and began to draw a circle, explaining that the circle was kind of like me. (1977: 426–427)

Harter then drew a line down the middle, putting an S for 'smart' on the left of the circle and a D for 'dumb' on the right, explaining to the 'teacher' that she felt dumb when she couldn't do her maths and smart at other times, like doing her workbook. The 'teacher' erased the drawing and continued the school lesson, but about ten minutes later, the 'teacher' reproduced the drawing and then explained with great earnestness to the imaginary class that the 'girl' (that is, the therapist) feels dumb and smart. "She feels both." The 'teacher' then used this concrete symbol over the next several weeks to represent different mixed emotions concretely.

In the above example, then, the child in therapy was repeatedly trying to integrate two personal schemas on a more advanced level. She had great difficulty resolving the schemas of 'smart' and 'dumb' into a more integrated and higher level schema. Unlike a younger and less cognitively mature child, this girl was struggling to move beyond a sequential level of emotional understanding. Before being able to do this on a purely internal level of mental activity, a concrete representation seemed to be necessary to aid her thinking. This process with affective schemas is similar to the concrete operations stage of cognitive schemas in which the child cannot operate on objects on a purely mental level.

The concrete symbolic representation aided both cognitive and affective understanding of these two personal schemas for this girl. However, it is important to note that this concrete representation was only one facet of the therapeutic situation. The circle was introduced at a critical point (the girl being 'stuck') of the therapeutic process; the child was allowed to make use of the therapist's representation spontaneously **in her own way**, without any pressure from the therapist to alter her thinking; and, finally, therapy was well advanced. The girl was able consciously to think about and recall these experiences of being 'dumb' and 'smart'; verbalization of these experiences was a common feature of the play sessions; and, finally, by adopting the role of the 'teacher', the child was simultaneously in a less threatening role than her own usual role and able to view objectively her own role from someone else's perspective, thereby reducing her egocentricity, as we shall discuss more fully in the concluding section.

Harter also illustrates the potential therapeutic mishandling of structured play experiences. That is, what was a useful symbolic tool for one child can be over-extended by the therapist to other emotional domains the child is not spontaneously exploring and over-generalized by the therapist to other children who might find this structure inappropriate. The aid then becomes a formal technique applied inappropriately with later children or overused with one child. Instead of being used to further a child's emotional understanding and his perceptions of personal experiences, it loses its impact and becomes more purely a cognitive device.

A non-directive play therapist, while making use of structured exercises, would only introduce them into the therapeutic situation tentatively and only then in response to an expressed or half-expressed need of the child. The following example may clarify this distinction.

Lucy began to paint a picture of the lion glove puppet. As she painted it became a teddy; a teddy who was a magician, with a magic wand.

> **Therapist:** And if the teddy magician could grant you three wishes I wonder what they would be?

Lucy began to paint again ... quickly and purposefully, she painted her two brothers whom she had been separated from when she was removed into care following sexual abuse (Plate 2). Her brothers had remained with her mother who was felt to be able to care adequately for the boys, as the father was now in prison, although the mother had been passively involved in the abuse of Lucy. Lucy viewed her two younger brothers as the only source of trusted love in her life. She was still desperate to be re-united with them although they had now been apart for two years.

In the painting Lucy was with her brothers and smiling – they meant love, warmth and the possibility of being happy.

She painted a second picture of a man behind prison bars, who she identified as her father.

> **Lucy:** I wish he could stay there forever. [In an angry voice].

> **Therapist:** And it's like he deserves to stay there.

Her third picture was a Christmas scene, with Lucy and her two brothers and their Christmas presents (Plate 3). Lucy talked about how much she wanted to be with her brothers at Christmas but her present carers had said they couldn't visit again because they were badly behaved.

ROLE PLAYING

Finally, we shall discuss role playing and the manner in which it emerges in both normal emotional development and within non-directive play therapy. A child can simultaneously achieve several different purposes through even very rudimentary role playing. A very common kind of role playing, and one which even a very young child initiates, is one in which the child takes the parental role. In doing so, and assigning the therapist his own usual role, the child can experience for himself what it is like to be his own parent. But in addition, the child is able to have a more objective view of himself. By distancing himself from his own role in this way, the child can view his own actions and feelings from the outside, a much easier task than trying to evaluate his actions and feelings while they are being experienced inside himself. The child, then, can simultaneously clarify his own actions and feelings from the outside, and internally experience and feel his parent's feelings and actions, at least in part, which he has previously viewed only from the outside.

These gains from role reversal happen in a child's spontaneous play. What makes the therapeutic situation most valuable for a troubled child who role plays is that as well as himself clarifying his feelings, thoughts and actions and, at the same time, his parent's corresponding ones, as he might do in solitary or group play with other children, he is now assigning the adult therapist a child's role. And while being in the child's role, the therapist is using her own feelings congruently. In using these feelings congruently, she is enabling the child to experience what a healthy and usual reaction would be for any 'child' in a similar situation. The child, then, is internalizing an emotional yardstick to use in judging his own similar experiences in the past and, perhaps, the present.

For example, Julie, age five, was sexually abused by her father, her principal caregiver, for two years, beginning at age three. The abuse had now stopped and Julie was being fostered by very caring foster parents. However, during the early sessions of play therapy it became apparent that Julie was very confused about appropriate sex role assignments. This was inadvertently compounded by the foster father calling Julie his "sweetheart" and his "girlfriend" in a teasingly affectionate way. In one therapy session Julie was playing with a Playmobil girl and gave the therapist a Playmobil man to use. The man and girl were playing together, sliding down a hill. The girl then said to the man, "come under here and kiss me under my knickers and then lie on top of me". The therapist, as the man figure[11] replied congruently that he was a man and he would never like to do that to a little girl. He could only do that with a big woman. But if Julie wanted him to be a man like that, he'd pretend to be. Julie didn't reply but made the man figure lie on top of the girl figure. She repeated variations of this play at several points in the next few sessions and was then able to make the girl figure get angry at the man figure for sexually abusing her.

Role playing, then, enabled Julie to experience the abusive roles again, but this time with the feelings of the therapist used congruently and incorporated later into her own play. Another feature of role playing illustrated by the above example is that role playing is a very common and nonthreatening form of interaction for children, given that the child himself controls the activity. Indeed, much spontaneous play of children centres around playing out various roles. (Newson and Newson, 1979; Isaacs, 1933). Even an emotionally disturbed and frightened child often is able to role play in a rudimentary sense, albeit in a rigid and very basic way, without language, what is often at the heart of his problem. It is a unique expression of a child's personality and a way of sharing himself with the therapist. From the therapist's point of view, when a child role plays it will help her to empathize more fully with the child by taking on his role, in addition to the child developing a different understanding of himself.

Another feature of role playing is that it involves the child experientially. The child acts and reacts, feels and thinks, talks and listens all at the same time, without separating out these functions. It involves the total child: role playing is more real than talking about experiences. Feelings are experienced more intensely as the child partially (as in all imagined experiences with an 'as if' quality) becomes the person whose role he takes. In this way the child can understand and change his inner world as he begins to understand both the person he plays and the person (the therapist) he observes playing his own usual role. Role playing partially accounts for the child's at times sudden changes in behaviour during therapy. He can move towards clarifying his own feelings, actions and thoughts as well as those of the person(s) he role plays, enabling the child to become more empathetic and often more altruistic towards others.

Another dimension of role playing that it is necessary for the therapist to be aware of is the natural development of role playing ability in children. The role playing of young children is quite different in nature to an emotionally troubled child's need for the play therapist to be the child's mechanical reflection, as we will illustrate in chapter 4. A very rigid structure in a child's role playing can indicate that there is a disturbance in his ability to role play. Indeed one indication of therapeutic progress is the child's increasing ability to engage in role plays with more fluidity and encompassing more complex experiences.

For emotionally healthy preschool children situations and roles in their play are usually simpler, based on their everyday experiences; they are not, however, rigid. Scenes are often centred around activities such as eating, going to bed, etc. (see Isaacs, 1933, for examples). The roles, too, are less varied, often being exclusively parent–child roles. For the therapist it is sometimes more difficult to follow a preschool child's role playing and take the appropriate role than it is to follow an older child's lead, who usually gives more information to the therapist on the expectations of the role she is to take. With young children and with silent children it is important for the therapist to have a general working knowledge of young children's experiences, thoughts and feelings in order to try out roles given to the therapist by the child without the therapist needing any verbal instructions. It is usually correct to assume in these situations that the therapist has been put into the child's role. The child seems usually to be feeling powerless and threatened and can more easily role play opposite and less negative feelings. As we suggested earlier, it is also safer for the child in role playing the adult to control the therapist's actions and, in turn, keep control of and keep hidden his own feelings and actions.

Children are also aware of and utilize shared rituals in their symbolic play from a very early age.[12] Since many role playing situations are based on standard rituals shared by most adults with young children in a particular culture, a therapist by being consciously aware of these rituals will be more able to distinguish her role assignment with minimal cues. For example, in England when a child picks up a cup and says, "We'll have a nice cup of tea", he is most likely conveying that he (the child) is in an adult, nurturing role and probably the therapist is in the child's role. In addition, the child role playing the adult role feels that he is in the powerful role, able to correct the actions of the therapist (as child) if the therapist misinterprets her role. In the above example, if the child had a unique meaning for this situation which the therapist misunderstood, the child might be able to say, "You have a bottle, not that cup, silly."

This example, by the way, illustrates how the therapist is treated by the child in the play therapy situation often in the same way that the child would treat a companion. The child tends to talk more directly, without the respect and reserve usually given to an adult. The therapist might be taken aback and find the tone of the child disparaging (and indeed, it might be!) until the therapist is aware of **why** the child has this lack of respect for her adult position. While, of course, the therapist must always maintain her respect for the child, it is necessary for the therapist to assume in these cases that she is not the child's equal or superior in play. The therapist is being assigned a role, again, and it is more likely to be a subordinate one, especially with troubled children.

In role playing, as discussed above, the child, and especially the younger child, seems to find it easier to maintain the situation's personal meaning and personal expression of feelings, thoughts and actions than in other forms of communication. Younger preschool children also find it more difficult at times that older children to maintain role reversal, and sometimes slip back and forth between playing themselves and playing the other person. This instability seems to be due to the child using mental images for thoughts which are rapidly changing in his mind.

This characteristic of young children's thinking seems to be one of the reasons for the child's lack of concern over continuity between players, sequences and so on. The child becomes aware of and acts out some of the mental images. It seems natural for him, because of his more limited cognitive capacity, to shift actions quickly as he processes his thought, without being able to take into account the impact of his thoughts on someone else.[13]

While it is usual for young children to engage in role playing spontaneously in their play, it becomes less common as a child matures. By pre-adolescence it has become relatively uncommon, since the process of internalization of symbolic play into daydreaming has largely occurred (Walls, 1972). Just as with other means of individual expression, role playing can still be a more natural and satisfying mode of personal expression for some older children and it seems to develop more complexity in these children as they mature. While it is a capacity that everyone can engage in to some degree, certain adolescents, and preadolescents, given the opportunity, show great skill in devising compli- cated dramas with intricate plots. They assign themselves and the therapist a variety of multi-faceted roles and personalities.

In therapeutically using role playing, there are certain skills which the therapist needs to develop, as well as having a knowledge of child development and cultural roles. The therapist working with younger children must develop the flexibility of mind needed to shift roles quickly with minimal cues. The therapist must also be able to take the child's inferior role without feeling too threatened by this loss of dignity. Also, in working with older children who are adept at role playing, it is very useful to have some acting skills, such as the ability to mimic and to act out a variety of subtle emotions. In addition, the therapist needs emotional resilience. The therapist needs her own role of therapist clearly in mind, and a confidence in herself, otherwise she can lose herself in the roles she plays. She also needs the emotional resilience to switch emotions quickly, even when these emotions seem incompletely expressed. Because role playing involves both the child **and** the therapist in a total sense, the therapist herself will naturally feel affected by the roles she is assigned and the roles and emotions the child is portraying. Acting out a role involves building up a whole set of shared understandings on a symbolic level, "(adults) are not just humouring children when they play with them like this; they are themselves affected by the power of the symbol." (Newson and Newson, 1979, 103) It must be recognized, then, that both the child and the therapist are affected by the symbolic power of role playing situations and this sharing changes and deepens their therapeutic relationship to one another.

Having discussed the theoretical foundations on which non-directive play therapy is based, we now consider in the next chapter the decisions which need to be made in setting up therapy with the child, demonstrating how these are informed by our theoretical understanding.

NOTES

(1) Rogerian non-directive therapy and Axline's non-directive play therapy can be classed as organismic theories (see Hall and Lindzey, 1978) and thus will be seen to be compatible with the developmental theory described here.

(2) 'Affect' will be used as a class name to include 'feeling', 'emotion', 'mood', 'temperament'.

(3) Affect, it is assumed, gives cognitive activity its interest and value; cognition gives highly affective activity, such as love, its aspects of understanding and judgement.

(4) Since Piaget's writing, there has been increasing emphasis in infant development research on precursors to 'deferred imitation' as well as on how social interaction contributes to the development of language and thought (see Stern, 1985; Hickmann, 1986). Examples such as David in chapter 7, section 3 and Jeffrey, chapter 6, point to a much earlier evolution of this process.

(5) This use of mental images has important implications for the ability of young children to testify to personal experiences and is largely unexplored in 'the child as witness' literature (see Ceci et al., 1987).

(6) 'Condensation' and 'displacement' are **not** used here solely to connote defence mechanisms, as they would be in psychoanalytic thought.

(7) See Reflection, chapter 7, section 1, for a discussion of the timing of these verbalizations in order to maximize communication and rapport with the child.

(8) Note that the therapist does **not** attempt to fulfil the child's more basic need for an attachment figure he can safely depend on in his everyday life (see chapter 3 on suitability of play therapy).

(9) More recently there has been a focus on the contextual determinants of a child's language rather than on his ideal competence. These functional models blur the sharp distinction between competence and performance of earlier models (Hickmann, 1986).

(10) For this reason, it is important that the therapy room be equipped with materials that are at a more advanced level of a child's cognitive development, as well as at a less advanced level (see chapter 3).

(11) See chapter 6 on gender issues in play therapy. The female therapist here was assigned a male abuser's role.

(12) See Newson and Newson, 1979, for an explanation of this development based on the playful interactions which develop between a baby and his mother.

(13) This is also characteristic of a child's recounting of a story or film (see Flavell et al., 1968).

— 3 —

Planning Decisions and Tasks

The following chapter deals with the decisions and tasks to be undertaken before engaging in therapeutic work with a child, and the issues which need to be explored at the beginning with the child, carers, and where relevant the referring agency. We conclude the chapter with suggestions for introducing the first session, this being the final point concerning which detailed planning decisions can be made before therapy with the child begins.

There are two stages in planning therapeutic work with a child: the first involves more general decisions about whether it is appropriate to undertake work with a particular child; the second more detailed planning, and negotiating an agreement with the child, family and agency.

We have ordered these decisions so that one can see what needs to be decided and worked on early, what depends on what, and what decisions taken at the first stage may need to be reviewed in the light of new or expanding information.

We recognize that although this implies that decisions are conscious and deliberate, not all planning will have this character. Although some decisions may be based on explicit thinking, others may be the result of a well-internalized practice wisdom, a feeling that 'this seems right'. However, particularly for the beginning practitioner, an investment in planning is necessary, and makes it more likely that the work will be successful and errors avoided.

INITIAL PLANNING

Decisions at this stage form themselves into three groups: the first concerns the child, and whether the nature of the problem makes it seem likely that he can be helped by individual work, and if so how long a period of help seems indicated; the second the nature of the referral; and the third, the situation of the therapist, and whether what she can offer is likely to meet the child's needs. As we suggested above, some of these decisions are interdependent: it may be for example that the child is appropriately referred, but that the problems presented seem likely to be too complex for the amount of time on offer. The order in which these factors are considered will vary too: sometimes awareness of a particular child's needs may prompt the therapist to do some initial planning; sometimes practitioners themselves wish to engage in more 'child-centred' practice and start actively to seek an appropriate child with whom to work. It seems right however to start with the child.

DECIDING WHETHER OR NOT THE CHILD'S NEEDS CAN BE MET BY INDIVIDUAL THERAPY

A preliminary decision needs to be made, usually before seeing the child and/or carers and on the basis of discussion with the referrer, as to whether the child can be helped by therapy. One cannot assume that individual couselling will be good for all children under all circumstances, and certain minimal criteria need to be developed.

On the whole there are very few problems experienced by children which could not in principle be helped by using this approach. Children who are extremely unruly and out of control, those at the other extreme who are withdrawn or experiencing a high degree of anxiety, and those whose lives, although on the whole stable, have been thrown into temporary crisis perhaps as a result of their parents' divorce, are all suitable. Some short accounts of children we have worked with may serve to illustrate this.

Gary was twelve years old when first referred. He had lived with both parents until he was five years old, when they separated, following which he spent many months going backwards and forwards between father and mother. From his mother he experienced rudimentary but ineffectual care, and was left alone in the house or to wander the streets for long periods. His father was physically violent to him, hitting and punching him for minor misdemeanours, and Gary always appeared cowed and apprehensive in his presence. At a routine examination at school, he was found to be sore and bleeding round the anus, and it was discovered that he had been subjected to anal abuse by his father from an early age. Following this, he was received into care, and experienced a succession of foster placements, all of which broke down because of his aggressive and violent behaviour towards the other children. When he was finally placed in a children's home, he attacked members of staff, broke the furniture and threw things at the other children, as a result of which he was kept locked in his room for hours at a time. Previous attempts to help him had included a plan based on behaviour modification principles, which had however appeared to increase his desperate outbursts of temper. He was referred as something of a last resort, in an attempt to control his manic behaviour, and the therapist felt that she could help him become less driven by his feelings, and less frightened and angry. He responded quickly, becoming reportedly calmer and much less disruptive, and establishing a close bond with the therapist.

Sara was nearly six years old when referred. She presented behaviourally and emotionally as a much younger child. Her speech was delayed and she found it difficult to relate to her peer group and adults, although there had evidently been an improvement in recent months in every area of her functioning. Despite this there was continuing cause for concern: she remained enuretic at nights and most days, she still occasionally soiled and had periods when she seemed deeply unhappy. Her concentration was poor, and she seemed isolated in her misery.

Sara had lived with her parents and two younger sisters until she was four years old. Her parents then separated and she had had virtually no contact with her father from then onwards. Some months later her mother, who suffered from deep bouts of depression, asked a cousin to care for Sara until she felt in a better position to cope. Sara was living with this relative on a voluntary arrangement between mother and cousin at the time of the referral. She was taken by the cousin to see her mother and sisters regularly once a week, and although apparently still wanting to see them, became painfully sad and forlorn after the visits. It was considered that therapy would help her resolve her pervasive feelings of sadness at the disruption, amounting to virtual loss, of her life with her immediate family. Over the weeks of play therapy, she repeatedly played out the themes of separation and displacement, using dolls and two dolls houses, until one day she finally shut three dolls up in one house, placed the fourth in another and said "Good-bye now" with a deep sigh and moved on to some different toys. Although continuing to have periods of sadness, she became generally livelier and more cheerful, and eventually became firmly attached to the cousin and her family, visiting her mother and sisters only occasionally.

Scott was eight years old at the time he was referred, to see if he could be helped to resolve his very confused feeling over his mother and his relationship with her. He and his two sisters had been received into care and placed in different foster homes after his elder sister had disclosed that one of her mother's boyfriends had sexually abused her. There had been a number of previous incidents involving bruising to Scott and one of the girls, but although there had been concerns about these, Scott had always denied that the injuries were deliberate. On arriving to stay with the previously unknown foster family, he announced that he wanted to return to his own mum "sometime but not yet", poignantly reflecting his uncertainty about her. He had got on well with an earlier boyfriend of his mother's, and was able to form an attachment to the foster father, to whom he subsequently disclosed that his mum had played "rude games" with him, and "sucked his tail in the bath".

He seemed to be much younger than his chronological age, with poor concentration, and played and spoke more like a five year old. He was treated kindly by his new classmates, but like a small pet rather than an equal. The psychic energy involved in keeping conflicting feelings at bay, and the anxieties about his mother and boyfriend had left him with little to spare for normal developmental tasks, and the experience of being helpless in the face of dangerous or disturbing behaviour seemed to have limited his capacity for growth.

His confusion concerning his feelings for his mother quickly emerged in therapy, and his behaviour gradually became more age-appropriate, reflecting a greater understanding, mastery and confidence. After a year in the foster home, and sixteen play therapy sessions, he successfully moved to a new adoptive home, where he settled well.

Beth was seven years old at the time of referral. Much to the consternation of her parents and school, she had become electively mute when she started primary school two years before, and her condition had remained unchanged since then despite speech therapy.

Beth was the middle child of three girls and was said to have had a normal emotional development in her preschool years and to have related well to her parents and siblings. Her parents told the therapist that Beth's introduction to primary school had coincided with the death of her grandmother to whom she had been very close and that she had since then refused to speak at school. At home Beth only permitted herself to whisper, even when she wanted things.

In ten sessions of play therapy, she progressed with marked rapidity, beginning to speak in a normal voice at home after three sessions, and subsequently beginning to communicate at school. She remained a somewhat shy and anxious child, but continued to develop normally.

A common thread running through the lives of all the children described above is that they are struggling to resolve feelings to do with loss, to establish a sense of their own integrity and ability to master events which have at times threatened to overwhelm them.

It is clear however that the experiences which they have to resolve, and their capacity to do so, are quite different. Beth, for example, seemed from the referral to be a child who although a rather vulnerable personality had been functioning adequately until her grandmother's death, and the hurly burly of school life created a crisis for her from which her own resources seemed insufficient to enable her to recover. Scott, on the other hand, although apparently having formed reasonably secure early attachments, had experienced prolonged emotional, sexual and physical abuse, but not the successive rejections which had been meted out to Gary.

This issue, of how seriously damaged the child appears to be, is one to explore with the referrer, since it is relevant both to the amount of time which the child will need, and to the experience of the therapist. We know from working with beginning practitioners that it is common to wish to help the most damaged or needy children. This seems to be both from a desire to expend what is after all an appreciable amount of time where it is most needed, and also from a feeling that it may be easier to work with a child whose problems and needs are very clear and where improvement is likely to be most discernible. Pressures from the employing agency to undertake work with the most disturbed children are also often considerable.

This, although understandable, is mistaken. We do encourage beginning practitioners to select initially a child for example like Beth, who is experiencing a temporary crisis, or problems in one area of life such as school, rather than the more damaged child. Gary's history of prolonged instability and rejection for example, make it likely that he will be extremely defensive and unable to trust. Helping him to get in touch with, and express what he is feeling is therefore much harder and is likely to take much longer than with a less damaged child. It is, apart from anything else, difficult for a worker who cannot draw on the experience of successful interchanges, to have the confidence and patience to wait out what may be a considerable number of sessions without anything apparently 'happening'. The temptation to direct the child to areas which one would predict are critical for him or her may become irresistible.

Another question to explore with the referrer is the current circumstances of the child. The child may be in a highly unsatisfactory placement, or shortly to be moved, or be in a situation where for some other reason a great deal of the child's energy will need to be channelled into merely surviving, or into defending against continuing negative experiences at home. Occasionally, as we indicate in chapter 6, children who have been sexually abused are referred for help even while they continue to live at home with the alleged perpetrator. In these circumstances, it is important to be clear that play therapy cannot provide a protective function and will almost undoubtedly be ineffective. Furthermore, the releasing and self-directive effect of the therapy makes it possible that in the short term the child's behaviour could deteriorate and become harder to handle: a withdrawn child, for example, who has been repressing angry feelings, may, feeling freer, begin to express them at home and sometimes at school. The setting obviously needs to be able to cope with this change in behaviour and in extreme circumstances (where the abuse for example is continuing), therapy could in fact place the child at greater risk.

Since therapists are often under pressure to provide help because of the very lack of stability which we suggest is a contra-indication, it is worth noting that our view receives widespread support in the therapy literature. Wolff, for example, argues that

We need to be clear that the last and most effective task [that is, reflecting back the child's communications] can only be undertaken when children enjoy real security in their lives. An eight year old who has lost two parents and whose temporary foster home is about to break down cannot possibly face his grief and fury, however skilled his therapist, until new parent figures have made a permanent commitment to him. He needs all the defences he can muster, even if, to preserve a cheery front, he has to soil or steal. (1986: 236)

In one instance, it was clear from the initial (agency) referral, that the carers barely tolerated their nine-year-old foster child, and that a different placement would need to be found. They seemed unlikely to support any change in the child and the start of therapy was delayed until she was in a more supportive setting.

Often, of course, the decision is finely balanced, a compromise between the neediness of the child and what could be achieved in better circumstances. Julie, age seven, was referred because of severe behavioural problems at home. The origin of her problems seemed manifestly to be located in the volatile and often violent relationship between her parents, in whose battles Julie became embroiled. She fiercely supported her mother, who would reject Julie as an ally when she again became reconciled with her husband, twice demanding that Julie be taken into care. Family therapy had failed to halt this destructive cycle, and the key worker had begun to consider initiating proceedings to remove the child on the grounds of emotional abuse, although still unsure whether there were sufficient legal grounds for doing this. While this uncertainty continued, it was clear that Julie needed help in making sense of her intensely angry feelings towards her father and protective uncertainties with her mother. It was equally clear that her parents would only support therapy on very limited terms, and could not be recruited to back up the therapist's work. It was decided nonetheless to go ahead with play therapy, because of Julie's needs and because a move in the near future seemed at best unlikely. The risk to Julie of exacerbating the situation for her at home was acknowledged, and the key worker undertook to intensify his involvement with the parents to minimize this.

Not infrequently, children are referred who become the subject of court proceedings during the course of their therapy. If these are imminent, then it may be advisable to delay the start of therapy until a decision concerning the child's future has been reached by the court. However (although this may change with the new time frameworks of the Children Act), the timing of court proceedings is notoriously unpredictable; moreover, it is often not clear at the outset of therapy that court proceedings will take place, and indeed they may be instigated partly as a result of what emerges in therapy. Where therapy is taking place at the time of a court hearing, it can provide help for the child, particularly by offering a place in which anxieties about it can be explored away from those who are more immediately involved. While the therapist has to be aware that difficulties can arise, for example, the child may blame the therapist for a course of action taken by the court, on balance we do not consider that the fact that a court hearing is pending is in itself a bar to effective therapy.

ISSUES CONCERNING THE REFERRAL AND THE REFERRING AGENCY

A number of issues need to be explored which concern the motivation and timing of the referral and the support which will be forthcoming from the referring agency. It is unlikely that the children or adolescents will themselves ask for counselling, so it is important initially to explore with the referrer his or her expectations from the referral and commitment to the therapeutic work.

If the referral is from an agency, perhaps following a case conference recommendation, the agency remit needs to be clarified. Frequently, for example, the agency expectation is that the work will involve an assessment of the child (whether the child should remain with the present carers/ return home/has other as yet unidentified concerns which are contributing to behavioural problems) or a validation of an earlier disclosure/suspicion of abuse. Alternatively, the involvement of the therapist may be seen as a form of insurance policy, a means of protecting the child which obviates the need for regular work and active monitoring on the part of the key worker. While the concerns of the child should become clearer during therapy, and the therapy may serve some protective function, it is important to emphasize from the outset that making an assessment/validating information etc., is not the purpose of the intervention and may or may not emerge from it. If, after discussion, it becomes clear that this is the agency's expectation, then a different approach, structure and contract needs to be sought. If, on the other hand, an open-ended remit is acceptable, then decisions need to be taken about the kind of information which will be fed back to the agency. Usually this will take the form of a report summarizing the work, with some evaluation of what has been achieved: we discuss this in more detail in the next chapter, mentioning it here because it may need to be considered briefly at this stage.

A not dissimilar process needs to be undertaken if the referral comes from a parent, care-giver or school, since again the expectation may be of something quite specific, for example that a particular behavioural problem will be worked on (for which usually read 'resolved') or something that appears to be troubling the child clarified. Again, it is important to be clear that although these issues may emerge during therapy, the agenda is for the child to determine and the work may take a different focus. The question as to whether or not it is appropriate in these circumstances to offer some kind of feedback of a general nature subsequently to the referrer is a complex one and will be discussed in a later section.

Implicit in this is the need, from the first referral, to begin to assesss why the child is being referred and whose problem it is. Something which may be perceived as likely to be difficult, or behaviours which are experienced as problematic by concerned adults, may not in fact be so for the child. For example, the children and adolescents who are referred for counselling have often experienced sexual abuse. Although this is likely to be identified as the reason for therapy by the referring agency, it may not be the most significant issue for the child. A girl of fifteen, removed from home after she disclosed abuse by her father, and facing life in a hostel after the breakdown of a subsequent foster-placement, spoke of the experience thus:

> **Rosa:** What my dad did wasn't so bad. He's a loving, he's a nice man, he's been a good father to me. After I'd been raped [by someone else] I couldn't stand it any more. I couldn't go on so I told. That was a mistake. I wish I hadn't.
>
> **Therapist:** Lots of good memories about him. Feeling it couldn't go on but regretting you told.
>
> **Rosa:** That's it, because now I've lost my mum. I can manage on my own all right [lip quivering, on the verge of tears] but I've got no family now. [very quietly] I've got no one.
>
> **Therapist:** Feeling you've lost mum, lost everything.
>
> **Rosa:** [Angry] I have, and he's got my family. He's got my mum and my brother.
>
> **Therapist:** He's got what's really yours.
>
> **Rosa:** And I'd do anything to get back. If he and mum would only say there was a bit of a problem and get some help, I'd be able to go back. I'd like to have him as my dad again. I do love him.

Here the trauma for the child is the loss of her family: Her need for her parents, her desire to get back into the home, and the pain of separation, rather than the feelings engendered by the sexual abuse, were for her the current critical issues to be explored.

One further aspect which needs to be addressed with the referrer is that the question 'who is the behaviour a problem for?' may suggest that some other form of intervention is more appropriate. Although this may not always be apparent until after contact with the family, social workers will be familiar with the situation where the child is being required to 'carry' what is in fact a family problem. For example, in one family where the child was initially referred, it became apparent that the problem lay more in the parents' competing claims and contradictory parenting of her and that work with the child on her own would do little to remedy this. The couple were referred to Relate, with an agreement that work would focus on their handling of their daughter, since they were, initially at least, reluctant to discuss their own relationship. In some circumstances, too, it may be appropriate for work with the child to be undertaken concurrently with other intervention in the family system. (See Glaser and Frosh, 1988, chapter 7, for a useful discussion of selecting different therapeutic approaches.)

Finally in discussions with the referrer, it is important to clarify from the outset that the roles undertaken by the therapist and the key worker are very different, and that because of this they should not be invested in the same person. In addition, when therapy is being offered by a practitioner from the same agency, confusion can arise as to who has responsibility for management of the case, and the co-ordination of the various aspects of intervention. It is also understandably tempting for a hard-pressed key worker in a busy agency to relinquish certain tasks to the therapist and the latter may therefore need to clarify from the outset the boundary of her involvement. Responsibility for co-ordination needs to be clearly allocated to a named individual, usually the social worker, who is aware not only of progress in the therapeutic work, but maintains responsibility for decisions concerning case conferences, court applications, communicating with school and carers and so on. Since some of the confusion seems to arise from a genuine lack of understanding of the nature of the therapist's involvement, it is sometimes helpful to clarify this in writing in advance of undertaking the work. (See appendix 1 at the end of the section for an example of a possible statement that may be used.)

ISSUES FOR THE WORKER

Making an internal commitment to working with the child

Starting therapeutic work with children is in a sense no different from undertaking any other form of planned intervention with clients. All require a commitment to regular sessions over a given period of time, properly supervised, monitored and recorded. However, it seems necessary to reiterate that for a child to benefit from therapy he must be able to trust in the worker's dependability over appointments. The working climate in which many practitioners operate unfortunately seems to tolerate or even encourage unplanned work, for example, a social worker, embarking on therapy, took an eight-year-old boy who had been placed in voluntary care by his mother, and then had experienced two foster home breakdowns, to see the play room where, he explained, they would be seeing each other regularly. A month elapsed before he next made contact, by which time, unsurprisingly, the boy declined to go with him.

By contrast, a twelve-year-old boy had been having therapy for a number of weeks. At one session, the social worker arrived half-an-hour late, having been delayed in an accident. The boy rushed out to greet her, seized her hand and said, "I knew you'd come for me. They said you wouldn't, but I wouldn't go till you came."

Sometimes when one has embarked on a particular piece of work, one becomes disheartened by lack of progress, settles for less than one had initially hoped for, feels overwhelmed by other demands on one's time, or for other reasons begins to doubt whether the expenditure of time and effort is worthwhile. However, one has made the commitment, and to withdraw prematurely is to risk further damaging the child, or replicating earlier experiences of breakdown of care. If personal circumstances seem likely to intervene, it is therefore better to make the decision not to go forward with the intervention before contact has been made with the child and/or the carers. This critical decision about engaging in therapeutic work can best be made on the basis of an understanding of the special characteristics of the approach, one's own work situation, and some awareness of one's personal aptitudes and tolerances.

The work setting

One should be in a position to offer a minimum of eight weekly sessions to the child at the outset. Although occasionally the child does not require this amount of time, or decides not to continue, offering less than this makes it likely that the work will either not get off the ground or be interrupted at a critical phase. As we indicated earlier, a very deprived child is likely to be highly defended and will need more time before he is able to trust enough to share well-hidden feelings, so that eight sessions is likely to be inadequate. The process too is likely to take longer with a less experienced therapist, who will be slower to pick up cues and to go below the surface content of what is being communicated. Having said this, therapy over an eight-week period does offer children, particularly those who are less traumatized, opportunities to work on their feelings.

Although possibly not so critical in this as in other kinds of work (for example groupwork can be effectively sabotaged by unsupportive colleagues) it is wise and proper to enlist the help and support of colleagues where possible. One therapist discovered just before the beginning of a session that her doll's house had been given away by a colleague to another client. Such behaviour might possibly have been avoided by prior discussion with the rest of the team concerning the nature of the work being undertaken.

Personal issues

We have already referred to some of the strains which this way of working may present for the worker who is more accustomed to adopting a problem-solving, decision-making way of working and would stress the need for deliberate and ongoing reflection on one's personal attitudes and experiences, particularly relating to one's childhood. It may also be worth exploring at an early stage, if one is undertaking this work for the first time, whether the age or gender of the child has any personal significance. Some practitioners find that they have a strong initial preference for working, say, with a boy from a pre-school age group. Although one should reflect on the basis for this (perhaps it arises from a sense of familiarity with one's own sex, or having children of a similar age) it seems sensible at the outset to follow an instinct for something which will feel more manageable. From the child's point of view of course, the gender of the therapist may need to be considered, an issue which we consider in detail in the chapter on working with children who have been sexually abused.

At this point in the planning, then, some preparatory work has been undertaken, but no promises have been made and no expectations raised. At the end of these discussions, the therapist should have explored the following issues, many of them with the referrer:

- Why the child is being referred (the nature of the problem and what it is hoped that therapy will achieve).
- Whether in addition to the stated objective there is any hidden agenda on the part of the referrer which would jeopardize the work or create a conflict between therapist and referrer.
- From the referrer's account of the child's problems, how long-standing and deep-seated these appear to be.
- With the answer to this question in mind, what appears to be the minimum number of sessions that the child is likely to need, and whether the therapist has the necessary time available.
- Whether the therapist both can and wishes to make the investment of time and energy with this particular child.
- What support will be available from colleagues.
- What support will be forthcoming for the child from his or her carers and school, particularly if the child becomes more self-assertive or vulnerable as more of his feelings surface in therapy.
- Whether the timing of the therapy is appropriate. If the child is likely to be moved, whether or not this is imminent, and, if so, whether or not therapy would provide support and continuity during this period, or whether it is better left until the child is more settled.

APPENDIX 1: STATEMENT CONCERNING THERAPEUTIC WORK

I have been asked by ... to consider working therapeutically with John, the eldest child in the ... family. Since I have not yet discussed the background details with the key worker I have not decided whether in my opinion therapeutic work is suitable for him. If I do agree that he would benefit from therapy, I would be able to begin working with him in September.

I normally offer twenty sessions of non-directive play therapy. At the end of the first ten sesssions, my practice is to review therapeutic progress and decide jointly with the child, if he is old enough, whether ten more sessions is appropriate. With most children referred to me, who tend to have long-standing problems, I usually think twenty sessions is a reasonable estimate of the time needed for effective therapeutic work, and request funds at the outset for this number. However, I also feel a review after ten sessions is helpful therapeutically, so that the timespan does not seem too long to a child, and so that the child can have some personal commitment to more sessions or, instead, decide that ten sessions is enough. At other times a child can make more rapid progress than anticipated, or his circumstances may change, and ten sessions is the maximum needed. I assume that the social worker for the family will inform me of relevant events and changes in circumstances of the child that may affect him therapeutically.

In addition to the child's sessions, I have an initial visit with the foster carers and/or the parents to introduce myself, explain the method of therapy I propose, ask for their co-operation and answer any questions they may have. At times during my therapeutic work with a child, a matter may arise that would seem to warrant a visit from me, rather than the key social worker, such as a possible breakdown in support from the family for continued therapeutic work or a request from carers or the social worker for insight into the child's behaviour and its management. I do assume, though, that my primary role is for the child, and not for the whole family, which is the social worker's responsibility.

I also visit the child's carers, usually towards the end of the requested number of sessions, in order to make an assessment of therapeutic progress and to make decisions about ending my therapeutic work with the child.

At the end of the sessions, I write up a general report on the child's therapeutic progress. I also write up a final report when the child's therapy finishes and submit them both to the social worker. These will be included as part of the sessional work and will not be separately invoiced.

S E C T I O N   T W O

FURTHER PLANNING

In the previous section, we considered the initial thinking and discussions that needed to take place before making a preliminary commitment to working with a particular child. On the assumption that this has been made, we now consider the further and specific planning decisions, which have to do with issues such as making a contract, deciding on venue, time-scale, recording and so on. A number of these decisions have to be made, and as before, many are inter-dependent. In addition, decisions taken at an earlier stage may need to be revised in the light of further information about the child and his or her family setting.

The further planning decisions to be considered here concern:

- What further information might it be desirable to have about the child?
- What physical setting will best suit the child one intends to work with?
- How should the playroom be equipped?
- What will be done with constructions made by the child in the session?
- What is the appropriate number and frequency of sessions to offer the child?
- For how long should each session go on?

- What time of day will best suit the child?
- What agreement about confidentiality is to be reached and what contact or communication maintained with the referring agency and/or the child's carers?
- What records should be kept for the agency and for the worker's personal use?
- What preparatory work should be undertaken with the child and carers?
- What supervision should the worker seek for support and for developing skills and understandings?
- What means can be chosen for monitoring and assessing the work undertaken?
- What further arrangements need to be made about the session?
- How will the first session be started?

We shall consider these points one by one, making links between them where appropriate, and assuming that issues to do with the initial referral have been worked out, and that the therapist expects to begin working with the child in the near future. The above decisions need to be considered in relation to all children with whom one is undertaking therapy. One further issue however needs to be considered in relation to many, but not all, of the children referred. Evidence of abuse, hitherto unsuspected, may emerge during the course of therapy, and practitioners need to consider their position in advance of starting the therapy:

What should the therapist's response be if a child makes a disclosure of physical or sexual abuse during a therapy session, or there are other indications that the child may need protection?

Although this question should properly be addressed in the planning stage the issues involved are complex and for convenience we consider them separately in a later chapter (chapter 7, section 3)

What further information about the child is it desirable for the therapist to have?

From the initial referral, the therapist will need to have gleaned enough information about the child's current circumstances, presenting problem, and history to be able to make a preliminary decision about therapy. Often further information, from the school, health visitor or the child's file is available, and consideration needs to be given as to whether or not it will be helpful to obtain it.

Certainly a working knowledge of the significant people in the child's life, their names, and critical events in the child's experience to date can be invaluable. Where, for example, there have been a number of people with whom the child has been involved it can be inhibiting and tiresome for the child if the therapist has to check out who the particular person is each time someone new is mentioned. Furthermore, knowing that the child has experienced care from stepfather, foster father and natural father can help one make better sense of what the child is communicating through a particular piece of play. A point reiterated in this book, and by other writers on non-directive play therapy (Axline, 1947; Moustakas, 1953) is that it is unnecessary for the therapist to know the 'real' meaning of the child's play – indeed, the attempt to understand it in terms of an objective reality may impede the recognition and reflection of the child's feelings which are being expressed through the play. Nonetheless, an understanding of the dynamics of the child's home and school life can sometimes help one to discern themes and reflect feelings with greater accuracy. This is probably particularly the case for the beginning therapist, for whom it is harder to make sense of what is happening, or who may lack confidence in having accurately identified the child's feelings. For example, a social worker new to this method of working was surprised when the child, having asked her to choose which of two figures should be the good one, proceeded to bury the good figure vigorously and aggressively in the sand, eventually using the bad figure to throw it to the other side of the room. The child's case file indicated that his behaviour was constantly contrasted with the 'good' behaviour of his stepbrother and sister. Although the therapist's reflection of the child's feeling had been appropriate, confirmation of the probable underlying dynamic helped her to respond when this theme again emerged fleetingly in the child's play.

The disadvantages of information sharing and file reading need also to be recognized. Children and adolescents quite understandably feel uncomfortable, vulnerable and sometimes angry that information has been shared about them without their permission. Sharing with the child the brief overview the worker has of their lives can be helpful and may dispel some of the fears or anxieties they have.

Having access to the child's file also carries with it the danger that the child has been proscribed before any personal contact has been made. Children as well as adults are often presented months, even years later, as they appeared when they were initially assessed, often at a time of crisis. A description of the child as aggressive, delinquent, immature, sexualized or withdrawn may be part of a snapshot that remains with the child as long as the record continues to exist, even though the child himself has changed.

Since it is easy to overlook medical problems as the reason for disturbed behaviour it is important to have a general familiarity with common medical problems, and to be open to the possibility that symptoms may be the result of an underlying medical condition. Assessment by other professionals may be essential in ensuring that the child does not have a physical illness or infection or in ruling out alternative hypotheses. For example, enuresis or encropesis may be indicative of a urinary tract or bowel infection; behaviour problems may be attributable to an undiagnosed hearing problem, and so on.

An educational psychologist's assessment is helpful where there are concerns about learning difficulties – lack of concentration or poor achievement may or may not be the result of trauma. Sometimes such an assessment may indicate that special teaching, or transfer to a different school or class is a more appropriate intervention, and that the child's behavioural difficulties are related to frustrations associated with inappropriate expectations of his performance. Sometimes the assessment merely indicates the possibility of a learning impairment. For example, Samantha was base-lined by an educational psychologist when she was moved from what appeared to be an abusive home environment into a foster home. At seven, her reading ability was non-existent, her speech poor, her sentence formation and vocabulary limited and her articulation made her difficult to understand. Her number work was also at a level expected of a much younger child. However, her mother had also had learning difficulties and had attended a special needs school, and her speech was still sometimes difficult to understand. Her father was also of low ability. Because of the parental history, the educational psychologist was uncertain about the level of Samantha's potential achievement.

Eight months later, having experienced a compensatory foster placement and weekly counselling sessions, she was achieving in school at an age-appropriate level in all areas. There was a marked improvement in her speech, vocabulary, reading skills and number work. The difficulties had it seemed been the result of the deprivation and abuse she had experienced at home.

Other professional assessment and intervention may also be necessary in order to support or supplement therapy. Rebecca, for example, age fifteen, was referred because she seemed unable to come to terms with the abuse which had occurred in her foster home some years before. However, alongside the regular counselling sessions she required medication to combat the clinical depression she was struggling with.

What physical setting will best suit the child one intends to work with?

We take this planning decision next because although it may need to be altered in the light of what later becomes known about the child, it is helpful to have given the question of venue some thought before going to see the child and family.

We recognize that the resources available will vary widely for different practitioners, and would make the general point that although the physical setting should be carefully considered it is not an overriding factor, and lack of optimum surroundings should not of itself be a reason for foregoing therapy.

This having been said, it is of course very much easier to work in a setting which is properly designed and equipped, and where the therapist does not have the additional anxieties of transporting toys and equipment on each occasion. It is important therapeutically for the child that the setting is familiar and consistent, and this is harder to achieve, as well as being time-consuming, if one is having to move furniture and equip the room from scratch for each session. Working in an unfamiliar setting, or one which is not home territory, can also impose additional anxieties which distract from the therapeutic work. It is hard enough, even in a familiar setting, to think through all the small decisions about limits which may arise during a session – does it matter if the child wants to paint the wooden easel? Will the clay come off the carpet? Will the next worker using the room mind if the puppets are damp? and so on. The need to balance the therapeutic use of limit setting with a reasonable respect for shared property is made more difficult in a setting where you are the guest, and the limits to acceptable behaviour are unknown (but likely, you suspect, to be stricter than your own).

Ideally, one would like to have a medium-sized room, sound-proofed, with a sink and toilet adjacent, in a setting which does not carry for the child negative connotations or stigma. It should offer privacy, be free from interruptions and be available each week for sessions with the child. It needs also to be a room where the child feels able to express himself as freely as necessary, and where the worker does not have to be preoccupied with protecting the furniture or floor from water, paint and clay.

The room should be furnished with part carpeting and part with some floor covering which is easy to clean; a table, some chairs, an armchair, a clock, an easel and two or three large pillows or bean bags. A sand tray, or a small plastic bowl for sand is useful. It is also helpful if water is available in some way either in or near the room as water play is a useful and expressive aid for play. These items facilitate the child's play, allowing him to sit or lie on carpeted floor and to splash water or sand on to the uncarpeted space. A table surface is necessary for a variety of the child's activities, the pillows can be curled up on or jumped upon, and as Kezur puts it, "the armchair comes in handy for the occasional cuddle" (1981: 8) as well as providing the possibility of distance for older children.

The size of the room has an effect on both the child and the therapist. A large room can be intimidating, even for older children and adolescents. Although it can offer advantages of space, in that a very active child may feel hemmed in if the room is too small, the therapist may find it difficult to keep up with the child and can feel rather overwhelmed by the activity going on. On the other hand, the child may need to be able to create his own private space, away from the scrutiny of the therapist, and can feel vulnerable and exposed if there is insufficient room for this. Often, too, as he begins to feel comfortable the child will make more use of the space available, and if this is too restricted, will be unable to experience the sense of increased freedom.

A seemingly confident twelve year old, for example, appeared to find a large purpose built play room very inhibiting. Not until the third session did he feel comfortable enough to begin hesitantly to explore the room. He did this by tentatively rolling marbles further and further away from his chair and then scuttled across the room to retrieve them.

The therapist also needs to identify a place in the room where she can sit, so that, particularly in the early stages of therapy, the child knows where she is, and is not startled by unexpected movements, or a sense of the therapist intruding into his personal space.

Soundproofing is desirable but rarely available. Others may complain about the noise the therapist and child are making – whether laughing, crying, singing or shouting – and come in to do so, or peep in to see what is happening out of curiosity. In the same way noise from others in the building can be intrusive and dispel the private character of the session.

Linda, for example, had reached a point in the fifth session when she was able to share and explore painful and angry feelings about her life. The staff meeting next door became louder as time went on, with much laughter filtering into the room. Acknowledging this to the child can sometimes be sufficient, although in this case the worker decided that it was better to interrupt the session and go and do something about the noise rather than to allow precious time to be invalidated by the intrusion.

Even very young children may be aware of the need for privacy, and it is necessary to think through the therapeutic implications for each child in relation to this. Some children may be very worried about not being able to get out of the play room, associating doors being shut with punishment, while others ask for the door to be locked. A child may also show signs that his therapy is reaching an end by becoming more interested in opening doors, noise outside, than he was previously.

Tina aged seven, who was being counselled in a room at a children's home, tried each week to lock the playroom door to stop children walking in. Each week she failed and asked the therapist to lock it. This continued for six months until finally, after much struggling, she managed to lock the door herself.

She turned round quickly, a wide smile on her face, and exclaimed with excitement, "I did it, I did it. I locked it. I locked it and no one can come in. It's our special time. It would make me feel sad if anyone came in."

Not all doors can be locked, and as adults and children often ignore notices hung outside, where privacy is an issue a simple wedge under the door is easily transportable and usually effective.

Children and particularly adolescents, can be sensitive to the windows in a room, and the possibility of being overlooked:

Rosie (aged fifteen) asked for the curtains to be drawn when she became aware of the window cleaner outside. "I'd feel stupid if anyone saw me in here with all these kids' things." She moved on to play with a doll and then set up shop, but was still clearly inhibited by sounds of the window cleaner outside, despite having the curtains drawn.

It may of course be the therapist who feels uncomfortable:

John (aged three and a half) was having his session in a room at his nursery school. The worker had been unaware that the windows in the room looked out on to the hall. Suddenly during the session twenty or so children's faces were pressed against the windows. The child continued to play unconcerned and absorbed, but the therapist, feeling as if she was working in a fish tank, was thoroughly disconcerted.

Lynn (aged nine) had reached a point in the session where she had begun to re-enact the abuse using the play materials available. She began to moan and breathe heavily. A colleague walked past the room and glanced in through the glass pane in the door. He went on and then came back and stood looking in, clearly anxious about what was going on. The therapist had to struggle with feelings of self-consciousness, although the child again remained absorbed in what she was doing.

As the above examples illustrate, lack of alternative resources sometimes makes the use of other than a properly designated play therapy room inevitable. If this is the case, it is important at the very least to try and ensure that the setting chosen will not be one that offers additional inhibiting factors for the child. For example, on one occasion, the therapist conducted a play session with the child in the child's foster home. It soon became apparent that the child was conscious of the foster mother's presence next door and found this inhibiting, even though the session itself proceeded without actual interruptions. (It later became clear that the foster mother in question was extremely punitive towards the child, making her self-consciousness very understandable. Although this could not have been anticipated from the referral, it does highlight the desirability of choosing a neutral setting in which to undertake the work.)

Very occasionally, there are circumstances in relation to a particular case which may indicate that a child would benefit from being seen on ground with which he or she is familiar. In the case of a disturbed three-year-old boy, for example, with whom his mother was desperate for help, the sessions in a regular play therapy room set in a pleasant social services building proved overwhelmingly frightening. It was decided to hold the first sessions in the little boy's home, with his mother present for part of the time, the familiar surroundings providing the reassurance he needed before he could begin to trust the worker and the process of therapy.

How should the playroom be equipped?

The kind of play materials and toys with which the room should be equipped will to some extent depend on the particular child and his problems and may become clearer after the therapist has met the child. However, there are certain principles on which the choice of materials should be based and certain factors to be considered when making the selection. Some items are used consistently whatever the age or gender of the child; the inclusion of others may depend very much on the age of the child, and to some extent therapists also develop their own preference for particular toys. We consider first some general principles in relation to the choice of materials, before discussing specific suggestions in more detail.

In general, the toys and equipment in the room should be sufficient to provide the child with the appropriate means through which to express mood and feeling. They should extend the age range of the child at either end, so that the child is free to be as young or as old as he wants. They should in the same way offer the child the possibility of playing with toys not usually associated with his or her gender. And they should on the whole encourage the use of the child's imagination, creative expression and feelings rather than emphasizing structured activities which tend to absorb the child's attention in completing a task.

It is unlikely that all the materials will be utilized by the child and a balance needs to be achieved between providing enough to allow the child free expression, and too much, which may clutter up the playroom and prove a distraction, particularly for a child who is very disorganized or has poor concentration.

Materials must also be carefully thought out in advance, since introducing new materials during ongoing sessions can create problems and draw a child to or away from a specific area of concern. For example, introducing water into the setting may give the child the message that the therapist finds it important for him to play with it, and can sidetrack him from freely directing his thinking in order to try and comply with the adult's wishes. Similarly, a preponderance of one kind of material rather than another may inadvertently convey a certain message to the child — for example, a large supply of cuddly toys may suggest to the child that largely affectionate responses are being looked for.

Moustakas, in a discussion concerning the selection of toys, considers the value of different kinds of play materials. Pointing out that sand, water, paints and clay are among the most useful items, he argues that:

The unstructured nature of these materials makes it possible for the child to use them in a way that enables him to express and release tense, pent-up feelings ... [they can] be deformed, amassed, spilled, spread, molded, combined, torn apart, brought into shape, or destroyed. It is also possible for the child to organize the material in such a way that significant interpersonal situations are recreated. (1959: 7)

Sand, water and clay are often initially useful in engaging the reluctant child, since they are less likely to be freely available at home. Toys such as guns, knives, swords etc. are frequently employed by children to express hostility, and may be particularly useful because children can use them to express strong aggression in socially acceptable ways. Animals are often used by the child to convey basic emotions, which may be less frightening to represent symbolically than through the more direct use of play figures.

In general, as we discuss in detail later, the child will play with non-threatening toys at the outset, and as sessions continue, will move into more intimate emotions, progressing from toys which are in a sense at one remove to more personalized toys and activities (for example, puppets or dressing up).

We do not want to be prescriptive about what is used, since this is an area where people develop different ideas, but particularly as practitioners may need to purchase some of these items or bring all the toys and equipment to the room, it may be helpful if we discuss items which we consider essential or desirable.

1. A good stock of plain white paper, preferably in at least a couple of sizes, wax crayons, felt tip pens and paints are indispensable. The room may not have running water, and even if there is a tap close by, it is useful to have water to hand in a flask or bottle. (This can be used for painting, giving dolls little drinks and so on.) We usually have an easel and paints, two or three broad paintbrushes, and a couple of fine brushes, used especially by older children.

2. At least one, possibly two dolls houses. If the playroom is having to be equipped from scratch each time, then one dolls house is certainly sufficient. However, two give the children more scope to enact significant events, moves or visits and one of the houses can become school or hospital and so on. Although slightly larger individualized houses may offer more scope, the Fisher Price type of house is perfectly adequate. Shoe boxes can also be used, among other things, as houses.

3. Dolls and cuddly toys. A set of the small pipe-cleaner type dolls are ideal, as they are pliable and children find them comfortable to hold and play with. They can be fed, put to bed, bathed etc., rather more easily than the Fisher Price plastic figures, and the different figures in the sets lend themselves to being various characters. Some sets include black and Asian figures. Failing this type of small doll, the Play People figures are reasonably satisfactory, and useful because figures representing different settings such as hospitals are available – although these are not essential since children will invent, and adapt what is there.

Other small figures, such as those from Star Wars, are adaptable, and can be picked up cheaply second hand at school fairs, toy stalls etc. Some children enjoy the type of Russian doll which conceals other smaller ones, and the type which consists of the larger doll containing half a dozen matched size smaller ones lends itself particularly well to symbolic play.

It is helpful to have one or two larger dolls, with some kind of wardrobe and equipment for beds etc. Some of the larger kinds of pliable figures, such as the old style action men, are particularly useful for boys, since they are free from the usual gender associations of other dolls, and boys can dress them and play with them with fewer inhibitions.

Some soft toys are useful, particularly the kind which can be used as hand puppets and provide a way for the child to communicate indirectly. Finger puppets also serve this purpose well. (However, small children, that is, under about the age of three, may not have reached a cognitive stage which enables them to makes sense of puppets, and can find them confusing.) Again, soft animals may provide boys with the opportunities to re-enact nurturing or caring activities in a gender-acceptable manner.

4. Clay/playdough. Both kinds of modelling material should be available if possible, especially for older children. It is now possible to purchase a type of clay which does not dry out so quickly and is therefore more durable. However, not all children like the feel of clay, and find playdough, or something similar, more acceptable. We usually make some dough, using a recipe familiar to many

playgroups, which is cheap and easy to make in generous quantities. It needs to be kept in a plastic bag between sessions, or it will dry out.

5. Sand is, as we suggest above, useful, but because it is difficult to transport and inevitably gets spilt, may be impractable for many settings. Since it provides the ideal means through which the child can work through hostile emotions (burying figures repeatedly for example as the little boy, G, described above did with the 'good' figures) it is worth thinking through what else might offer this instead if sand is unavailable.

6. One or two children's books, colouring books, jigsaws and puzzles are helpful, either for when the child is wishing to 'coast' rather than engage in free play, or is tired, or for offering a means of shared activity. A disadvantage of these, apart from the risk of structuring activities too much, is that they may encourage the practitioner into pursuing the game for its own sake, rather than holding on to the focus of its meaning for the child.

7. Anatomically correct dolls. We explore the use of these more fully in a later chapter but in general have mixed feelings about including them routinely. Clearly they can be useful, and occasionally the child's play with these dolls can clarify the fact that sexual abuse has taken place. It is possible that they may assist the child in getting in touch with feelings about a particular abusive experience, perhaps by indicating that subjects relating to genitals and sexual bodily functions are not taboo. On the other hand, children seem easily capable of adapting what is available in order to make the desired communication. One four-year-old graphically demonstrated what her father had done to her older sister, using two of the He-man series of dolls, He-man and Sheba, to do so.

Furthermore, some children, particularly older children and adolescents, can find correct dolls threatening and/or embarrassing and children's reactions to them can be varied and are not always predictable. Our tentative conclusion therefore is that unless the therapist is confident in using them appropriately and is relatively familiar with the child's needs, they are inadvisable and should not be included routinely in the equipment.

8. Dressing up clothes. These do not need to be elaborate, but should include enough to allow the child to become, or to direct the therapist to become, a familiar or a fantasy figure. Hats (a policeman's helmet, fireman's or soldier's hat, a straw hat which can be decorated with scarves etc.) and jewellery are particularly useful. Cloaks, long dresses, a handbag, a military style jacket have variously been pressed into service.

9. A plastic tea-service. The ceremony of tea is deeply embedded in many cultures and the ritual of having a cup of tea seems to offer endless opportunities for such themes as giving and withholding, sharing, having/not having enough and so on. One small, deprived eight-year-old drank voraciously from the teapot spout, holding his hand or a puppet to his cheek as he did so, only gradually moving to drink from the baby's bottle as he became more able to trust the relationship with the therapist.

10. A baby's feeding bottle. Many (although of course not all) children of any age use the bottle for comfort and the re-working of earlier experiences and this should be included routinely in the equipment. The message that this item gives, in this kind of permissive setting, is that the child may, if he wishes, act younger than is appropriate for his age and work is often done with the child around this issue. It may be hard for the child to accept (and give himself) permission to feed from the bottle. Richard (age 8), for example, clearly curious about it, said scornfully that only babies drank from bottles. The therapist commented that sometimes children too liked to play with a bottle. It took four sessions of these tentative enquiries before he started to take small, surreptitious sucks from it, then curled himself into a large cardboard box and drank, only breaking off for the bottle to be refilled.

11. A plastic gun (preferably a pop gun which fires ping-pong balls), sword or dagger are useful, as we indicated earlier, for the expression of aggressive feelings, although predictably enough these tend to be used more by boys than girls.

12. Small farm animals, bricks and materials for building. Plastic or wooden snakes are often the focus of fantasy play, again often as a means of expressing aggressive or fearful feelings.

13. Small vehicles, such as cars, trucks, police cars and ambulances.

It is important to maintain consistency both about what the room contains and the way in which the toys and materials are set out. The more secure and familiar the child feels in the setting, the more he or she is freed to address deep-seated and often frightening feelings. The absence of a familiar item, or an alteration in the arrangement of the room may upset the child in a way that seems out of all proportion at a commonsensical level; although such an experience **can** be used therapeutically, usually it proves a disruption from what the child is working on.

Finally, it is important to try and see the play room through the eyes of the child who is to be worked with. With younger children, it is important to have materials within the child's reach, so that he can play with them as he wishes. Older children particularly may be sensitive to a room which suggests a much younger age and may need time with activities which they regard as more appropriate, such as painting, before venturing into other areas. Furthermore, many emotionally deprived children have to struggle to hold together an older identity and need to feel secure before they can gradually begin to let go of it.

One twelve-year-old boy, for example, for many weeks persisted in giving his age as two years older than it was, only gradually feeling able to relinquish this grown up self, and act as a much younger child. A sixteen-year-old girl played constantly with the dolls and dolls house, but was at a conscious level aware that these were for younger children and for a time became self-conscious if she felt herself observed by the therapist. When starting working with older children, therefore, it is helpful to set out the room with an emphasis on age-appropriate materials, paper, paints, clay, modelling tools, games and jigsaws for example, keeping the dolls houses, cuddly toys etc., in the room however so that they can gravitate to these if they wish and as they feel more comfortable.

What should be done with constructions made by the child in the therapy sessions?

We take this planning decision next because it relates both to the way in which the room is set out and to the way it is equipped. Thought needs to be given in advance about what to do with constructions, paintings, clay models, etc. which the child produces during his sessions. This can also extend to alterations which the child has made to the layout of the room. Some children specifically ask the therapist to save what they have done; others seem indifferent to things they have made. The therapist needs to think through two related issues here: first, what are the realistic limitations on saving the child's creations. Sometimes, this may restrict other children's use of the room, for example, preserving a clay model may mean that no clay is left for others. Some rooms have boards on which children's drawings can be posted, but leaving other children's drawings on it can sometimes prove a distraction for a particular child. In general, it is not possible to save materials which restrict other children's use of the room, and this may be even more the case where the room is also used for purposes other than play therapy.

The second related aspect to think through is the therapeutic implication of responding to the child's wish to preserve things he has made or, equally, his indifference to what happens to them. We explore some of the underlying feelings (for example, a difficulty in sharing) which these reactions may suggest more fully later. It is worth noting here, however, that it seems important for the therapist to be responsible for those articles which can be kept, perhaps by saving them in a folder which can be mentioned at the appropriate time (sometimes towards the end of the time together, sometimes when the child asks or comments on what to with something he has made). In general, it seems right that the therapist should convey to the child that she respects what he does, but should also allow him to have his own feelings towards them (whether indifference, satisfaction or possessiveness.)

What should be the frequency, timing and length of sessions?

Decisions need to be taken in advance about the frequency and duration of each session, and the optimum time of day at which it will take place. The latter decision will need to be discussed with the child and family, but it is helpful to have given some thought to it in advance.

As Whitaker (1985) points out in relation to groupwork, the frequency with which sessions are held has an influence on the intensity of the experience for the client and the sense of continuity which can be established.

On the whole, the more frequently sessions are held, the more intense will be the experience and feelings generated by them, so that the ratio between the time spent in therapy and time spent elsewhere does affect the impact on the child. Thus sessions held twice weekly will have a greater quality of intensity than if they are held once a fortnight. However, one should not unquestioningly make the assumption that greater intensity is desirable, since for some clients too intense an experience can be overwhelming and can also get in the way of everyday activities. Moreover, it is clear that much work continues to be done between sessions on what has taken place within the therapy hour itself – indeed for therapy to be effective it is arguable that this process must take place. An interval between sessions may therefore allow this necessary assimilation to occur and re-affirm a sense of being in control. Oaklander makes a similar point when describing the child's use of a game at the end of a session as a way of saying: "Let's stop now. I need to assimilate what happened, allow for integration, mull this over." (1978: 172)

Another factor to be taken into account is the age of the child. Younger children have a very different sense of time from adolescents or adults and may find it more difficult to maintain a sense of continuity and for the momentum of one session to feed into the next if the intervals between the sessions are too long.

For older children and adolescents therefore, we suggest that weekly sessions offer the optimum balance between intensity, continuity and the assimilation of the experience. With younger children (under four or five years) it may be worth considering twice weekly sessions as optimum. However, we recognize that for many practitioners, such frequency may not be feasible, and successfully work with children as young as three years on a weekly basis.

For how long should each session continue?

Therapists from different theoretical frameworks show remarkable consistency in regarding an hour as the optimum length of time for each session to last. Much shorter than this, and the child may have had insufficient time to find and explore a particular theme: much longer, and the session becomes less focused and the intensity lost. If the therapy is being conducted properly, then the work is demanding both for the child and therapist, and it is difficult for either to maintain the same level of concentration and to continue to use the time fruitfully for much more than an hour.

Sometimes at the beginning of therapy, or for young or very damaged children a shorter time, for example thirty to forty minutes, proves enough. We discuss ending sessions in a later chapter – suffice it to point out here that the possibility of negotiating shorter sessions, either in the pre-planning stage or after the play therapy has started, should be borne in mind.

Whatever the length of time negotiated, the length of the session should be agreed with the child in advance (with a younger child perhaps showing him on the clock when the session will end) and the length adhered to. It can sometimes seem difficult not to extend the session, particularly when it seems that the child is in the middle of something important, and to cut off at this point will stop this flow or seem rejecting. However, the establishment of a time boundary is critical: the child learns to recognize it, and can use the time to limit or keep control himself of the extent to which feelings and material are explored: unlimited time can, paradoxically, reduce the child's ability to lead the session. A clock should be kept in the room, and the child alerted to the ending of the session ten minutes beforehand for an older, or a few minutes beforehand for a younger child.

Children cannot always manage the whole hour, and it is necessary to be sensitive to their wish to leave. Particularly at the beginning of therapy, the stress may be such that the child can only manage a short time to begin with and it is helpful to alert the carers to the fact that the early sessions may be somewhat shorter and to ask them to wait for the child in case the session ends early. Equally the child may experience something outside the session, or during it, which makes it painful to continue. One child, for example, who had asked to be taken into care a few days earlier and was still in a disturbed state of mind, found it difficult to enter the play room. Reflecting this feeling of uncertainty, the therapist suggested he might like to come in for a few minutes but that he could go or stay as he wished. The child opted to stay for fifteen minutes and then go. It is important to convey to the child that the session can be concluded when he wishes. Opinion varies as to whether or not to state this as a ground rule at the beginning of therapy, or to wait and address the issue as and when it arises. The latter is probably more appropriate with younger children, for whom a lot of verbal information unrelated to their actual experience at the beginning is fairly meaningless and difficult to remember.

Should the therapy be open-ended or time-limited?

In general, in all forms of individual and groupwork, the usual advantages of a time-limited structure are seen as allowing clients to take the fixed number of sessions into account and pace themselves accordingly, and enabling both clients and worker to concentrate their efforts and make better use of the time than when it stretches indefinitely before them. Setting the limits of time communicates an expectation that much can be done in the time available, and encourages people to act accordingly. An open-ended commitment however takes into account that, particularly with very damaged or deprived individuals, it may be impossible to predict how much time is required, and communicates the message that the therapist is ready to offer support for as long as it takes to work through the difficulties.

We do not see much advantage, however, in offering a long-term but time-limited intervention. A time-length of, for example, over six months, is difficult for the child to grasp and is unlikely to carry much meaning for him or her; it is unlikely therefore to encourage focus or pacing, and since the amount of time required is so hard to predict, will not greatly assist the therapist in planning.

Often, as we suggested in the previous chapter, the therapy will be constrained by the limits on the worker's time, which need to be explained to the child. The therapist must be aware of the restrictions that this imposes on the kind of work which is undertaken, and consider in advance the impact on a damaged child of breaking off the therapy when much remains unresolved and the child still has much to gain from the intervention.

As a general rule, we find it preferable to offer a limited number, usually of ten sessions to begin with, with the promise of a review and the possibility of a further ten afterwards. This has the advantage that the child has a say in the commitment to further work, and the agency has some clarification in allocating resources. One child mentioned earlier, who was very reluctant to engage in therapy, was offered six sessions initially, and the therapist committed the time to the child, whether or not he chose to come. Six sessions clearly felt more manageable at the outset to this particular twelve-year-old, who was able to choose for himself at the end of the six weeks that he wanted to continue for an open-ended number of sessions.

At what time of day should the session be held?

One should try to choose a time of day when the child is not too tired to engage and concentrate, at the same time as causing as little disruption to the child's school day as possible. By about eight or nine years, children are still fresh enough to be able to benefit from a session immediately after school and a small packet of biscuits and drink can be provided to tide them over until teatime. If they are younger than this, we try to see them during school hours; if the child is worried about missing school, it is usually possible to find enough time in the lunch hour.

What agreement about confidentiality is to be reached and what contact maintained with the referring agency and/or the child's carers?

Issues of confidentiality are particularly problematic for those working in the field of child abuse. In all therapeutic work with children, therapists will need to consider what communication to establish with the child's carers and what kind of information concerning therapy to share with the referring agency if there is one. In addition, therapists working in both statutory and private settings are bound by a code of ethics in relation to child abuse which requires them to share information concerning abuse with the statutory authorities concerned. Even though the firmly established purpose of therapy is to counsel the child rather than for example to provide evidence in court proceedings, therapists need to address such issues as to how they would respond to a child's disclosure of abuse, requests from the referring agency to provide evidence in court and so on.

We discuss some of the related practice issues that may arise in more detail later, but it is necessary to think out one's position broadly in advance of meeting the family and child. Although linked to this (since it concerns confidentiality) the keeping of records raises some different issues, and we consider recording separately.

The circumstances in which one may be asked to communicate information vary:

1. The child's parents or carers want some discussion during or at the end of therapy, in order to help their understanding of the child and give them guidance and direction in looking after him/her.
2. The referrer (assuming another colleague or agency) seeks some discussion during or at the close of therapy in order to help future work/planning for the child.
3. The carers (or school or others involved) report a deterioration in behaviour/increase in bedwetting/nightmares, and express concern about what is happening in therapy.
4. The therapist becomes concerned, on the basis of work with the child, that the child's needs are not being met in the current setting.
5. The child, in the course of therapy, reveals material which indicates that he has been abused.
6. In the course of therapy, material emerges which provides support for one course of action (for example removal from home) and the therapist is asked to provide evidence of this in court.
7. The therapist is asked to attend a case conference or planning meeting to give her view of the child.
8. The child requests the therapist to attend a meeting, for example a case conference, to speak on his or her behalf.

In all these situations, the need to put the best interests of the child to the fore is paramount: however, it will be evident that the decisions are not straightforward; for example, it is not easy to balance the need to try to ensure that the best decision is made for the child, by appearing as a witness in court, against the possible impact that the knowledge that some of the content of the session has been made public will have on the child.

There are however some general principles on which these decisions can be based. The responsibility to protect the child from harm is overriding: therefore should the child say or do anything which gives the therapist cause to think that the child is at risk, then this cannot be kept as a matter between the child and therapist and the information must be shared with the statutory authority so that a decision may be taken about possible protective action. Although practitioners in statutory settings may be more conscious of agency guidelines in relation to child abuse, this obligation to share information extends, as we suggest above, to therapists in both private and statutory settings. However, such unequivocal evidence of risk is often not forthcoming; more usually, the child says or does something which is suggestive, but no more, of abuse. There are a number of issues arising out of this, particularly concerning whether or not the therapist should move from a non-directive approach in order to clarify what the child is saying, and whether or not, should an investigation be proceeded with, a different practitioner should undertake the validation interview. We consider these in detail in chapter 7.

Where the ultimate responsibility for the child's welfare rests with the referring agency, or with the child's carers, then the requirement to share some information through a verbal or written report about the progress of therapy or to give evidence about the child's needs to a court is a legitimate one. In principle, this information should enable those involved better to exercise the responsibility for care of the child and a reluctance to provide this feedback fails to recognize this, or to acknowledge the nature of the therapist's responsibility to the agency or referrers. It is also desirable to avoid building up a mystique about the therapy which alienates those involved in the day-to-day care of the child, and may make them more inclined to sabotage rather than support what is being done.

However, the therapist still has to take a decision about just what information should be shared. Children have a right to privacy, and this becomes particularly important when their time with the therapist is being presented as their 'special time', and when so much of the therapy is directed towards helping the child identify and feel confident in expressing what he is feeling. A further concern may be felt by the therapist as to the extent to which children are able to understand what is at issue over confidentiality, so that the position may be experienced by the practitioner as ambiguous and possibly uncomfortable as a result.

Many children, particularly those in the younger age group, are untroubled about these issues, and spelling them out at the beginning can feel rather intrusive, as if one were following one's own agenda rather than the child's. On the whole, however, it seems wise to say something, however briefly, at the outset, because of the difficulty of it becoming an issue later on: the child may feel betrayed if nothing has been said initially.

It is worth noting too, that some children provide graphic illustration of the fact that they do make some distinction in what they are saying, and are aware of the external context. One child, for example, aged seven, drew a picture which she presented to the therapist, giving a list of all the people who were not to see it. Another, older child switched off the tape at a particular point, thereby indicating to the therapist, among other things, that the tape had introduced an element at least of uncertainty into the session – but also that the child felt able to switch it off when she felt it necessary to do so.

We usually, therefore, agree to give some broad feedback to agency and carers, but differentiate between the kind of feedback we give those with key worker responsibility for the child, and those concerned with day-to-day care. To the agency, we outline the themes which have presented themselves, and comment on what we see as the child's future needs, and likely difficulties. We explain to the child at the outset, briefly, that we shall talk to their social worker and describe how we think the child feels now, but that we shall not repeat the exact words or detail of what has been said or done in the sessions unless the child specifically asks us to do so. With the carers, if it seems appropriate, we might discuss general issues of management which the therapy sessions have suggested – for example, over issues of punishment, where the child seeks out punishment because it confirms his sense of worthlessness.

Sometimes during the progress of therapy, those involved in caring for the child request contact, perhaps because the child's behaviour has deteriorated, or because of other concerns, for example over a possible move for the child, difficulties over access and so on. Usually in these circumstances it seems helpful to visit the family/school etc., to discuss these concerns, to provide reassurance, encourage those involved to be supportive rather than punitive towards the child and so on. However, it is important to keep these discussions focused on the child and to keep them general rather than specific. The temptation may be to become involved in working with the family, for example, and in practice it can then become difficult to maintain a firm boundary around the work which is being undertaken with the child. For this reason, therefore, contact with the carers should be maintained at single, one-off sessions, and any on-going work undertaken by someone else, usually the key worker for the family.

On occasion, the therapist may feel that because of material which is emerging during sessions with the child, more immediate contact is needed with carers and/or key worker. For example, a nine-year-old boy, who had been in a foster placement for a year, began in therapy to indicate real distress concerning his foster father, and it became clear from the content of his play and what he was saying, that he was spending much time locked in his room in the evenings and at weekends. The therapist, with the child's agreement, and having discussed her concerns with the key worker, visited the foster home, and subsequently recommended at a case conference held at her instigation, that the boy should be moved. (This course of action did not, incidentally, prove acceptable to the key worker, highlighting some of the inter-professional difficulties which can arise when more than one worker is involved, and when one worker, who is more closely identified with the child, offers what can be seen as unpalatable information concerning the agency's planning for the child.)

What records should be kept for the agency and for the therapist's personal use?

A decision needs to be made at this stage about the form of recording which will be used. Therapists in statutory settings will need to meet their organizational requirements concerning written records, for which purpose a summary of the main themes of the session is usually adequate. Over and above this, practitioners should keep a record for their own use, to be kept in the restricted part of the file, in order to develop their understanding of the child and learning about their own behaviour and responses, to help them recall information which the child has given them, and to form the basis of any further reports or records.

For increasing one's own understanding, an audio or video recording of the session is invaluable; it provides a faithful record of what was said, pauses, tone of voice, making it possible to recover the sequence in which things happened, reflect on the quality of one's responses, and so on. Sometimes the affect of a session may make it difficult to recall, the child may be particularly vocal, the themes may alter with great rapidity: a number of reasons may make it difficult, even with training, to recall the session accurately. A contemporary record also serves for the protection of the therapist and for evidence in court proceedings. However, it is important to bear in mind that abused children may have been involved in making pornographic films, so that recording their sessions might carry for them painful connotations. It is also important to ensure that the necessary permissions for recording have been given, for example by the child's parents or the courts; and to bear in mind that a court may request that a tape recording, once made, be produced in evidence.

It should be noted that the position concerning the exact status of audio-visual material made for therapeutic purposes is at present unclear. While some attention has been paid to the status of tapes made for disclosure purposes (see, for example, Butler-Sloss, 1988: 209–212) far less has been given to that of the audio-visual records of other clinical work, and some of the ensuing problems (for example in terms of storage) should their retention become a requirement. As Bevan states in a useful discussion of the circumstances on which the local authority may claim immunity from disclosing **written** records, ''The courts have not attempted to catalogue the kinds of recorded information that may be protected.'' (Bevan, 1989: 15.107) In the absence, therefore, of clear directions from one's agency or the courts, a written agreement with those concerned, including, when it seems appropriate, the child, stating the purpose for which the recording is being made, who will have access to it, and that it will be destroyed when the work has been completed, should suffice, and seems consistent with the practice endorsed in the **Cleveland Report** in relation to recordings made during disclosure interviews. (Butler-Sloss, 1988: 212)

Since some of the interaction in the session will be non-verbal, a video recording is likely best to capture what has gone on; however, unless a room with a fixed camera is used, or the camera can be set up and operated with minimal fuss by the practitioner, then an audio tape is almost as good, although this may need to be supplemented by notes or sketches if the child has, say, drawn something with particular intensity. For the inexperienced therapist, it is useful to transcribe the tape as one is listening to it; this helps one to stay focused and concentrate on what is happening, and having the transcript also makes it easier to reflect on what was said, see how the child works and how you as the therapist respond, and to refresh one's memory before the next session. With greater experience, it may be sufficient to listen to the tape and make notes; in either case, with an audio-tape it is important to listen to the tape soon after the session, since as much of the session may be non-verbal it is easy to become confused about the sequence of play, etc. It also facilitates the work of the consultant, who is then able to comment in detail on the transcript.

It must be acknowledged that listening to and transcribing tapes is a time-consuming process; students on our courses are asked to set aside a couple of hours for recording each session. Although with more experience, it is usually enough to transcribe particular key passages, and note key themes or activities, listening to tapes and reflecting on them still continues to take about as long as the session itself. We are only too aware of the demands that recording in any fashion, let alone in this detail, makes on the practitioner and that it is not merely a matter of self-discipline but also of fitting this into an already pressurized working schedule: but although some streamlining of the process becomes possible with experience, it is difficult to do justice to the child and to develop one's skill as a therapist without this investment of time in writing up the work.

It is sometimes said by practitioners that clients will not agree to the session being taped, or would not agree if asked, or that it is unethical to ask children to allow the session to be taped because they are powerless to refuse and their agreement is therefore enforced. Although clients, adults and children, do sometimes object to tapes, or one is sometimes uncertain that they have given 'informed consent', in general this seems to happen infrequently. Usually a matter of fact request at the beginning of the session for permission to record it, "which will help me think about things you've said", clarifying that it will be heard only by the practitioner and her consultant (if applicable) will be enough. Other children may indeed welcome the recording, feeling that it sets straight what has been said.

Occasionally, as we indicated in an earlier example, children do object to the session being recorded. It goes without saying that this should be respected: if it seems appropriate to explore the feelings behind the reluctance, then the therapist must be clear that this exploration is not prompted by any ulterior motive of getting the child to change his or her mind.

In the absence of a taped record of the session, then process recording should be used. Although it can never of course be as accurate as tape, the discipline of recording sequentially does enable one to recall a surprising amount of detail, not only about what was said and done, but about the transitions, and produces a far fuller record than unguided recall. The process record should note not only what the child said and how the practitioner responded but also non-verbal responses, how the therapist felt about what the child was saying and so on.

Whether transcribing a tape or process recording it is useful to adopt the device of recording on two sheets of paper, keeping the left hand side for a log of what was said and done, and the right for recording one's impressions, interpretations and comments. The advantage of this method is, as Whitaker suggests, that it "can be difficult to discipline oneself to produce a descriptive log which is not coloured by personal interpretations and reactions. The divided page helps." (1985: 137)

Having written up the session in detail, it is useful to note certain aspects of it in particular:

- Points when you were/were not child centred, and what seemed either to help you to remain focused on the child's needs or to draw you away from them;

- Points at which your responses were: accepting or not, empathetic or not, congruent or not;
- Significant moments or statements by the child, for example where the child seems to move forward, or to begin to function in a healthier or more positive way.

Therapists vary as to whether or not they feel comfortable making notes during the session. It can be intrusive, and may momentarily interrupt one's focus on the child and extensive note taking is clearly to be discouraged. However, it can be useful to keep a note pad handy on which to write a brief **aide-mémoire**, even when the session is being recorded, if something has been said or done and particularly when a sequence of play might otherwise be forgotten.

Some thought, finally, needs to be given to the access that the child should have to the record. Most practitioners in statutory settings will now be bound by their agency's policy on access to records, which customarily gives the client the right to see the agency worker's records, unless it can be argued that it is not in the client's interest to see them. (See DHSS Circular the **Personal Social Services Records – Disclosure of Information to Clients**, which sees non-disclosure to clients as the exception rather than the general rule, but suggests that it may be justified, **inter alia**, in order to "protect provisional opinions and judgements which social workers may have recorded". (Bevan, 1989: 15.107)) Practitioners in other settings may not be bound by such policies, but still need to think out their position on sharing records with clients.

A distinction in our view needs to be made between sharing with the child who wishes to see them, the verbatim notes on the session, and sharing those parts of the record which contain the practitioner's hypothesis and feelings about what was occurring. The latter are by their nature speculative and may have a damaging effect on the child if seen, particularly in the practitioner's absence. It therefore seems ethically right to restrict the child's access to the verbatim record. If the adjacent page format described above has been adopted the child then has access to the verbatim account but not the therapist's speculative comments.

For example, Rita, a fifteen-year-old was being seen in therapy for the first time. She had a long-standing history of problems, having been abused by her stepfather over many years, and had received hospital treatment for enuresis. She was reluctant to take the prescribed medication to help resolve a recurrent urinary infection. The therapist noted in her record of the first session:

The smell of stale urine in the room, which was rather on the small side, well-heated and poorly ventilated, was rather overwhelming. Rita was stressed and uneasy at being with me. She was pale and sweating, and sat as far from me as the room allowed, with a table pinned in between us. She said she didn't know what I was going to do. How our time together would be. What was expected of her. I was very conscious of the smell throughout, and clearly this was something real, in the present, in the room, and something which needed sharing. I felt however unable to find a way of reflecting my feeling which would not seem cruel and critical when our time together was only just beginning.

Later in the notes she records:

The enuresis has caused Rita to be isolated from and sometimes bullied and jeered at by her peer group. Her stepsister and the school have forced her to take baths, but it seems that the pain of all this is less costly than the pay-off – namely, that she is less likely to be sexually abused – if you are smelly, you are less appealing.

Rita, reading these comments in the notes, could only have been hurt by them; and they were after all only a hypothesis, written to help the practitioner in her understanding of Rita's feelings. Although one might wish to consider the appropriateness of leaving this detailed record on file permanently when the work has been completed, ethically it seems that to withhold this from the child is proper and in her best interests.

What supervision should the practitioner seek?

The availability of practitioners who are willing and trained to act as consultants varies enormously throughout the country. Some workers will have supervision or consultation built into their work setting, others will be working in considerable isolation. It goes without saying that good supervision, which provides one with the opportunity to examine and reflect on one's practice, is an invaluable adjunct, not only for the beginner but also for the more experienced therapist. Although we are only too well aware of the difficulties in securing it, we should stress here that we consider it essential that beginning and inexperienced therapists should only practise under supervision.

Ideally one wishes for a consultant who is experienced in working non-directively with children, with whom one can discuss the appropriate selection of the child, explore the planning issues described in this chapter, and who will provide on-going supervision and comment on the transcripts of the sessions. In the absence of someone experienced in working with children, we would seek a practitioner who is familiar with working non-directively with adults, since many of the skills are transferrable. It is also important to select someone whose work and judgement one respects. Above all, it seems vital that the consultant accepts and and is ready to work with a non-directive approach: it may be alien to some practitioners, and if one is struggling with issues around emotional congruence and non-directiveness, it is unhelpful to be supervised by someone whose approach is interpretive, problem solving or behavioural.

What preparatory work needs to be undertaken with the child and the carers?

One should by this stage have considered most of the detailed decisions discussed in this chapter, and have identified those which may require further exploration with the child's family and possibly subsequently need to be reviewed with the key worker. Some preparatory work must now be undertaken with the child and the family. It is as well to bear in mind at this stage that parents may show a range of responses which lead one to question the efficacy of treating the child in this home setting: for example, they may show overt hostility to the child or a reluctance to co-operate with therapy. In these circumstances one may conclude that other kinds of intervention are more appropriate and more readily acceptable to the family.

It is proper to think through in advance of the interview what one is trying to achieve in it, since this will guide one's decisions about who should be present and what needs to be discussed. The primary concern is usually to make oneself known to the child and to the parents or carers, to explain what the therapy will consist of, to give information about the structure and timing of the sessions, and to seek the child and family's agreement to it taking place. Many parents understandably feel unsure or vulnerable at the prospect of professional intervention and discussing with them what will take place, issues of confidentiality and so on may serve to alleviate at least some of their anxieties and enlist their support for the involvement. In addition, the therapist should discuss what kind of contact the carers may have with her, seek their permission to audio or video tape the sessions and make detailed arrangements about such things as bringing the child for the sessions.

Some thought should be given as to whether or not one wishes to meet the family and child together first of all, whether to see the family first and then talk with the child on his or her own, or whether to arrange separate meetings. To some extent, this will depend on the age of the child. For example, David, aged three, was first seen at home with his mother, and the possibility of therapy discussed with both of them. David, who had been referred by his mother because of his violent outbursts against her, his six month old sister and stepfather, was eager to begin, presenting as a bright articulate child with a powerful role in the family. His mother was ambivalent, hoping that play therapy might remove some of David's more difficult, hostile behaviour, but anxious about what he might say. Having spoken with David, the therapist spent some time separately with his mother, exploring with her some of her reservations, and encouraging her to think through how she might respond if further difficulties arose. Because of the mother's anxieties, the therapist indicated that she would be ready to come and discuss these again if further problems arose during therapy.

In a preparatory meeting with a rather older child, the foster parents were fully supportive and positive about counselling. Tina, however, who was a tense, watchful, anxious little girl, was clearly worried about the prospect. The therapist spent some time with her on her own, and eventually decided to conduct the sessions initially in a playroom at the foster home, rather than attempting to see her in an unfamiliar setting.

Although such difficulties cannot always be anticipated, a joint meeting with both carers and child present can be problematic. For example, at an introductory meeting with Linda, aged eleven, and her foster parents, the therapist was introduced briefly by the key social worker who then left. The therapist began to discuss the nature of the counselling that she was proposing, and the structure of the sessions, but was interrupted by the foster mother, who said aggressively that most people in their position would not have a child like Linda living with them if they knew her background. Both foster parents proceeded to express strongly negative feelings about Linda who went very red and looked acutely embarrassed.

The therapist intervened, acknowledging the difficulties which the foster parents felt Linda presented them with, but commenting on how uncomfortable and upset Linda looked at hearing all this being said. She made it clear that she felt it inappropriate for this information and their feelings to be shared in a way which became damaging to Linda.

Clearly such a situation poses a dilemma for the practitioner. If one identifies with the adults to the detriment of the child, then this may adversely affect the possibility of establishing a trusting, empowering relationship with the child. If one allies with the child, then one risks alienating the adults, with whom the child has to continue to relate and live when the therapist has departed. In the case described above, by acknowledging the feelings of both parties, but making it clear that the foster parents' rather cruel and thoughtless comments were unacceptable, the therapist felt that she had to some extent retrieved a difficult situation. Although the foster parents looked somewhat taken aback, and seemed ambivalent about the sessions, they rather grudgingly agreed to the therapy, saying that it might help Linda create fewer problems for them. Linda continued to hang her head, but looked faintly relieved, and readily agreed to weekly sessions.

Younger children particularly, but sometimes older ones too, express anxiety or diffidence about attending sessions on their own. It is highly desirable for the mother, father, or whoever has the primary care, to bring the child to the first session. Quite apart from offering reassurance to the child, it underlines the appropriate parental task and helps encourage the adult's involvement and support. Jeannie, aged eight, initially asked if her younger sister could come with her, and join in the first session. The therapist considered that it would be more appropriate for Jeannie's mother to come, at least for the first session, feeling that otherwise responsibility for supporting the therapy would be shifted away from the mother, and also that the presence of a lively three-year-old would make the session somewhat difficult to handle.

It is helpful if the carer, having brought the child to the play room, can be encouraged to return within about half an hour and wait in the vicinity, since for many children the first session can be stressful, and a full hour may initially prove too demanding for them to last out.

What means can be chosen for monitoring and assessing the work undertaken?

We are conscious here of seeking to address in a short space a subject on which there is an enormous literature. It is however evident from the literature that along with the other therapies, with the possible exception of behavioural therapy, it has proved difficult in non-directive therapy to identify the appropriate as well as ethically acceptable means of evaluating its effectiveness.

We suspect that one of the impediments to evaluation has been a tendency to think of it in terms of the collection of quantitative data generated by behavioural methods. In addition, as Haugaard and Reppucci suggest (1988) many clinicians are rightly uncomfortable with the experimental manipulations that often accompany outcome research.

However, even when means of evaluation are used which do take account of the particularity of individual cases and are directed towards the collection of qualitative data, it may be hard to provide a clear enough baseline description or a statement of goals which adequately reflects the process of therapy.

For example, as we discuss in some detail in chapter 4, part of the therapeutic process may involve the child in moving from a generalized inhibition to the expression of specific fears; the child's behaviour may become more challenging or difficult to manage as he becomes more confident and freer in expressing himself; and further problems (for example relating to abuse) may emerge as therapy progresses. In other words, any process of evaluation must be able to take account of the emergence of new information as the case proceeds which may suggest the modification or abandonment of the original therapeutic goals.

Nonetheless, it does seem important to move towards a more systematic collection of data in relation to therapy, in order to be able to monitor and evaluate therapeutic services to children. Haugaard and Reppucci suggest, as an initial step, that "one way of providing valuable outcome data without using an experimental paradigm would be for clinicians to report their cases in the literature, specifically detailing the methods that they employed and their successes and failures". (1988: 375) The general sequence of thinking that is involved in the method of evaluation known as single case evaluation – formulation, hypothesis, intervention, evaluation and follow-up – does as Sheldon argues "represent a considerable advance on the ad hoc procedures presently in use" (1983:499) and can take account of such issues as the need to modify earlier goals, discussed above. (See Sheldon, 1983, for a fuller discussion of this approach to evaluation.) In addition to accounts of the process, interviews with schools and carers to establish the extent of perceived change in the child would also provide relevant information on the effectiveness of therapy.

What further arrangements need to be made?

Further arrangements usually concern such things as transport, room booking, confirming the appointment with the school, and so on, but it is useful to check this in relation to one's own situation. If at all possible, arrangements should be made for the child to be transported to and from the session by someone other than the therapist undertaking the play therapy. There are obvious difficulties about preparing and clearing up the room if one is also involved in transporting the child. A further problem can arise, in that the kind of contact one makes with a child to and from a session will be of a different order to the non-directive approach within therapy; although children do in fact seem to accept the switch readily enough, it can be harder for the beginning worker to do this and may make the process of establishing the appropriate therapeutic stance more difficult to work out. It is often possible to secure a voluntary driver, or a taxi with a regular driver with whom the child has become familiar is usually acceptable. It is important however to establish that the child does feel safe and comfortable with whoever undertakes transport.

How will the first session be started?

This is the last decision that the therapist can plan at leisure, because thereafter what is said or done in the session is in response to the child.

It is important to recognize that for the child, the first session can, as we have said above, prove stressful; over and above anything else, therefore, it may be helpful to have at the back of one's mind Axline's description of therapy as an "offering of emotional hospitality to a child", and therefore to try by one's behaviour and responses to convey both a welcome and an acceptance of whatever the child brings. This may include accepting the child's reluctance to be in the play therapy room with you, hostility, ambivalence and so on. Although with an unfamiliar child it is difficult to empathize with the accuracy which comes with greater knowledge and ease, some reflection of feeling, for example, "It feels hard for you to be here", a respect for and sensitivity to the child's caution or whatever is important.

It is often helpful to reiterate very briefly (assuming that therapist and child have already met) the reasons why you and the child are meeting, perhaps making reference to the child's social worker or whoever has referred the child and stating the length of the session and the number of sessions that are planned. With a younger child, it is helpful to point out the clock, and to show where the hand will be at the end of the session. With all ages, we explain that we shall tell the child when the session is near the end.

Therapists vary as to whether or not they introduce any ground rules at this stage, some preferring to explain that the only rules are that the child is not to break the toys or equipment, or hurt himself or the therapist. On the whole, it seems to us preferable to wait to state this until as and when the occasion arises. It is often difficult for the child to take in much at this stage; a long state- ment can impede the therapist from being receptive to how the child is feeling; occasionally, the statement can prompt the more disruptive child to put these limits to the test immediately or make a timid child more fearful; and finally, it is unlikely that these are in fact all the rules that have to be made. It is difficult to anticipate them all, because children test them out in different ways: and it arguably gives a mixed message to mention certain rules and not others.

We conclude this chapter with an extract from the first session with Gary, a small, disruptive eleven-year-old, who had been living in a children's home for the past five years; the placement was near to breaking point because of Gary's abusive and disruptive behaviour.

The residential staff were uncertain whether or not he would come to the sessions. He arrived at first in an angry mood. He didn't like the room, it was too far to come. If the worker was to see him at all, it would have to be on his terms. He'd only see her where he lived.

> **Therapist:** Angry about being brought here. Feeling we should meet at your place.
>
> **Gary:** I might be needed there, no one will know where I am, they won't be able to find me. There might be an important phone call that I will miss.
>
> **Therapist:** Being here you might miss out on something important, you'll be out of touch with what's going on. [He glared round at the paints, toys, etc.]
>
> **Gary:** I'm not a child. Back at ... there's a room to talk in. I don't want these toys.
>
> **Therapist:** It's insulting having toys and things in here. You're too old for these things.

Half-way through the session this view had altered. He began to explore the glove puppets. He was delighted with one in particular. He was smiling and relaxed and seemed momentarily a much younger child.

> **Gary:** It's really neat.
>
> **Therapist:** You really like that one ... like to stroke it.

The session ended with Gary ready to come back the following week.

4

The Process of Play Therapy

"What must I do to tame you?" asked the little prince.

"You must be very patient," replied the fox. "First you will sit down at a little distance from me – like that – in the grass. I shall look at you out of the corner of my eye, and you will say nothing. Words are the source of misunderstandings. But you will sit a little closer to me, every day ..."

The next day the little prince came back. "It would have been better to come back at the same hour", said the fox. "If, for example, you come at four o'clock in the afternoon, then at three o'clock I shall begin to be happy. I shall feel happier and happier as the hour advances. At four o'clock, I shall already be worrying and jumping about. I shall show you how happy I am! But if you come at just anytime, I shall never know at what hour my heart is to be ready to greet you ... One must observe the proper rites ..." (**The Little Prince**, de Saint Exupéry, 1943: 84)

We have already set out (see chapter 2) the theoretical basis for non-directive play therapy, discussing general assumptions about consciousness, the place of play within this general framework, and the particular role of play therapy in a troubled child's mental and emotional life. In this chapter we shall use an extended case study to incorporate these theoretical aspects and to illustrate the general process of therapy, demonstrating how this process is used by each child in a unique and individualistic way.

The chapter is divided into two sections: the first section considers the following stages in the process of therapy: first, setting up therapy sessions, including background information, venue and meeting with the carer; second, the initial sessions; third, the middle sessions, including a relationship of false independence, the development of initiative and mutuality, the development of symbolic play and the experiencing of self-controlled regression; and fourth, the final stage, including inner acceptance, normal play, and a shift in family dynamics. Each stage is illustrated using the case material of Helen, a six-year-old girl, followed by a discussion of specific aspects of her progress in play therapy.

The second section contains a general discussion of the process of play therapy.

S E C T I O N   O N E

AN ILLUSTRATIVE CASE STUDY

SETTING UP PLAY THERAPY SESSIONS

Background information

Helen, who was six years old at the time of referral by her school, may be characterized as a "borderline" child (Ekstein, 1966) who seemed to be nearing the point of psychotic breakdown. Prior to the referral she had been receiving intermittent psychiatric help, including drug treatment for hyperactivity and dietary restrictions. Despite this intervention, she was described by her mother and teachers as having become increasingly disturbed and 'wild': her behaviour took the form of frenzied outbursts of rage against the adults around her, lashing out, using taunting behaviour and language, and sometimes defiantly exposing herself by taking all her clothes off.

Helen was the elder of two girls, born to parents who later divorced and cared for since then by her mother. Her father had little contact with his daughters. Helen was described by her mother as having been a problem even as a baby; she had refused cuddling and went rigid when held in her mother's arms. Helen reminded her mother of the girls' father, by whom she had been beaten: "Helen always had the same expression of anger in her face." In contrast, Helen's younger four-year-old sister was regarded by her mother as "easy to manage, eating well and loving to be cuddled".

The physical differences between the two sisters were marked. While the younger sister was relaxed, smiling, physically well-developed and attractive, Helen was very thin, with protruding eyes, a taut body stance and a rigid facial expression (except for times when her face would change to an expression of glee, which would quickly be followed by mischievous or provocative behaviour). Both children attended a small primary school, well experienced in working with deprived and problem children and their families. The school had

---

a flexible programme which allowed attention to be paid to individual needs. Helen however was considered to be highly disruptive, with increasingly severe behaviour problems which were unmanageable by the school.

Discussion of Helen's background information

Helen was referred by her school after her mother had urgently requested help in enabling Helen to remain in school. As we discussed in chapter 3, the first decision to be made by the therapist was whether (given Helen's background information) it was appropriate to work with her.

An immediate question was whether Helen's problems had a medical foundation and/or whether intensive psychiatric treatment, rather than non-directive play therapy, would be more appropriate, given the severity and long duration of her problems. A psychiatric assessment suggested that Helen's problems had an emotional origin and would potentially be responsive to therapeutic intervention.

The next question was whether family therapy, or therapy for the mother, rather than individual work with Helen, would be more appropriate, since the background information indicated a longstanding breakdown in the mother–child relationship. The fact that Helen's mother had projected the father's characteristics on to Helen from infancy onwards suggested the possibility that she herself had a personality disturbance. Another likely family dynamic was that Helen was being scapegoated, and identified as the 'sick' one in the family in order to allow the mother and younger sister to maintain their 'health' (Satir, 1967).

Another possibility, given Helen's history of self-exposure, was that her sexualized taunting behaviour was due to sexual abuse or trauma, although no other information indicated this.

Helen's mother, however, had adamantly refused treatment both for herself and her second daughter, yet seemed desperate for help for Helen. Because of this, and because of Helen's increasing distress, a series of twelve play therapy sessions was initially offered, with the possibility of further sessions if the early sessions seemed effective.

As this and our discussion in the previous chapter suggests, to make considered judgements about the usefulness of non-directive play therapy, knowledge of both normal and abnormal development is necessary in order to assess how serious the problems described in the referral are. Some problems have a medical basis, while others are more suitable for psychiatric intervention. It is also important to have a working knowledge of family dynamics in order to judge whether play therapy is appropriate for particular families. In Helen's case it would have been desirable simultaneously to engage in family therapy or therapeutic work with the mother as well as individual therapy for Helen. However, since her mother refused treatment so categorically, accepting Helen for therapy seemed to be the only way the family would allow change to occur. In other cases, if there are stronger grounds for suspecting abuse by the child's family, or if the parents are unco-operative and block therapeutic work with their child, interventions other than play therapy would be necessary. It is essential to recognize in assessing a referral that, as we point out in chapter 3, in some cases individual therapeutic work can make the child's home environment **more** abusive and threatening to him.

Another consideration in working with Helen was the amount of time needed and available to the therapist for treatment. Because of the severity and duration of Helen's problems, it would have been unrealistic to expect significant change to occur in eight or ten sessions. Hourly sessions over a six-month period, on a weekly basis, seemed indicated. These sessions were offered in two blocks of twelve sessions each. (These concerns are also discussed in relation to general planning issues in chapter 3, to which the reader is referred.)

The venue for Helen's play therapy sessions

The setting for play therapy was carefully chosen to maximize Helen's sense of security. The school was co-operative and provided a room for therapeutic use which was private and adequate, with the advantage of being familiar to Helen. The adaptation of this classroom, rather than using a purpose-designed play therapy room at another venue was decided to minimize disruption for Helen and increase her sense of safety. The room was across the courtyard from her classroom, which gave her easy access to it and the possibility of having shorter sessions if needed. The room was medium-sized, with shelves and lino floor, and windows at medium height (looking onto an empty site) and an adjoining toilet and washing area. Toys were provided by the school, such as an easel and paints, paper, dolls house, furniture, and doll family, bricks, dressing up clothes and dolls. These were supplemented by the therapist with hand puppets, a toy gun, a snake, felt tips, pencil, baby bottle, tea set and baby blanket.

Meeting Helen's carer

The therapist arranged a meeting at school with Helen's mother. The therapist talked initially about her general approach to play therapy: she explained that children often find it easier to play out, rather than talk through, their problems; that in play therapy children can select their own toys and talk or not as they wish; and that the therapist is there for the child's benefit, to help the child sort out what he feels and thinks. Another point (which did not seem to be an issue for Helen's mother, but may be so for other parents) was that Helen would have a need for privacy about her time in the playroom. The therapist explained also that although she would keep notes on the sessions with Helen, it would be for her own records, to help her in her work, and would not be discussed with anyone else. Obviously, if something dangerous to Helen or to other children emerged in the sessions, then the therapist would have a duty to report it. But in general, if Helen felt a sense of privacy in the sessions, she would be more likely to think deeply for herself about what was troubling her and not be influenced by what other people wanted her to say and do. (See chapter 3 for a further discussion of confidentiality, including the recording of sessions.)

Another issue the therapist discussed with Helen's mother was that children often need more support, not less, while attending play therapy sessions. Sometimes a child changes, but in ways that for a time may seem worse to the carers. The child may have nightmares, may demand more attention, may become more clinging and babyish or start asserting himself more. The therapist also stressed that when Helen began to change, she would not be able to change all at once; the adults would need to be patient with her while she was learning to act differently. The ways in which she changed might suit Helen, but be difficult for her mother to accept initially, until the benefits to Helen could be clearly seen.

Helen's mother, while sounding desperate for help and promising her co-operation, still remained very uninvolved. She repeated several times that it was the therapist's job to try to help Helen and that she herself could not reach her. The mother also remained physically rigid throughout the conversation, with every movement carefully controlled. (Unlike Helen, her mother was meticulous in her appearance, speech and manners.)

In offering twelve play therapy sessions initially the therapist stressed that it would be a joint decision, if possible, between herself and Helen as to whether or not to continue for twelve further sessions. Helen's mother was also offered time with the therapist to discuss any general issues about children and childcare that might arise for the mother, with the therapist commenting that she would be happy to be available for the mother at any point during the therapy sessions with Helen.

The therapist concluded by discussing practical matters, such as Helen wearing play clothes that could be washed afterwards, the time of the sessions and their duration. On the way out of the building, the therapist showed the mother the room she would be using in the school.

Introduction to Helen

Before beginning sessions with Helen, the therapist was introduced to Helen by her teacher. Without talking directly to Helen, since Helen had turned away from her, the therapist briefly explained the arrangements which had been made for the therapy. She went outside during playtime and stayed in the background, observing both Helen and her younger sister, and also enabling Helen to scrutinize her from a distance.

The purposes of this brief introduction of the therapist to Helen at school were to familiarize Helen with the therapist, to set up the play therapy room for the following weeks, to introduce the staff to the therapist, to familiarize the therapist with the school and the teacher, and to observe Helen in her school setting.

Because the venue was unfamiliar to the therapist, time was needed to evaluate the therapeutic implications of the room. Having decided on the selection of toys and arranged them so that Helen would have easy access to them, the therapist needed to locate a set place as a base for herself in the room. While this was helpful to the therapist's feeling of familiarity in a strange setting, it was even more important to Helen, who would know where the therapist was without looking directly at her. Helen would also be more secure in knowing that she would not be approached without warning by the therapist or that she in her turn would inadvertently come too close to the therapist. Thus, Helen would be reassured by the therapist's stillness and would not be frightened by any quick movement or threat to her personal space (see Tinbergen and Tinbergen, 1983).

HELEN'S INITIAL PLAY THERAPY SESSIONS

The first three sessions with Helen were very difficult both for Helen and the therapist. The entire hour was spent with Helen moving from one part of the room to another and one toy to another, always in sharp jerks and completely silently. Helen carried out these fragmented actions in the area near the door, at the greatest possible distance from the therapist. In each session, after shutting the door, the therapist took a seat on a low chair in the far corner of the room. During each hour Helen approached the door several times and tried the handle, then hesitated and began her fragmented exploration all over again. Although Helen was totally silent, the therapist verbally reflected Helen's feelings at times during the hour. These comments were based on Helen's non-verbal behaviour and on the therapist's own feelings. Helen ignored the therapist almost completely during these initial sessions, keeping either her back or the side of her body turned towards her. The only point of contact made with the therapist was when Helen had the side of her body turned towards her and once or twice during each session, lifting her head, risked a fleeting, surreptitious glance at the therapist.

The first session began when Helen was brought to the playroom by her teacher. As Helen entered the room for the first time, the therapist explained that she was going to shut the door and sit in the far chair. Helen could play with anything she wanted in the room and that they had an hour together until eleven o'clock. As the therapist said this, Helen appeared very agitated, yet silent. After sitting down, the therapist quietly, with a gentle voice tone, remarked that it was hard to be in a room with somebody you don't know; then she remained silent.

After a few minutes of exploratory, jerking actions near the door, Helen tried the door handle for the first time. The therapist quietly said that Helen wasn't sure that she could remain. She had some time left to stay, but if she wanted to go early today, she could leave and come back next time. Helen seemed to change her mind and began exploring the room again. The therapist reflected this change, saying, "You think maybe you'll stay for a while longer." During each of these three sessions the therapist made other brief comments such as: "You want to leave and you want to stay at the same time"; "You don't know what to do here"; and "It's hard to stay and hard to leave." The therapist also occasionally made brief statements about what Helen was exploring in the room, but for most of the time there were long periods of silence.

By the third session the therapist felt that Helen was familiar enough with the therapist and the room to comment when Helen quickly glanced at her that Helen sometimes liked to look at the therapist and didn't want to be seen looking. She also reassured Helen that the therapist did not need to look at her if Helen didn't want her to. During the rest of the session Helen was able to glance more frequently in the therapist's direction, particularly when the therapist talked to her. Seemingly, she began to realize that she could trust the therapist not to intrude on her and that it was Helen's choice when to glance at the therapist.

In general, however, Helen's initial sessions were marked by an absence of any kind of play beyond touching a toy or an object near the door and then jerking to another object or back to the door. She spent most of her time standing immobilized, facing the door with her back to the therapist and her head down.

DISCUSSION OF HELEN'S INITIAL SESSIONS

Helen, because of her acute mental distress, exhibited extreme fear and distrust in her initial sessions. Great care was needed to create a trusting environment and to help her establish a relationship with the therapist. A stable environment was maintained for Helen by working in her school and ensuring that the playroom remained the same for each session. Even more important was the therapist's behaviour within this setting: voice tone, timing of remarks and movements are all vital in creating a safe relationship with the child. (See Tinbergen and Tinbergen, 1983, who discuss the importance of exceptional patience, tact and unobtrusiveness in observing animal behaviour and extend this to children with autism.)

With a highly anxious child like Helen, a quiet, gentle voice is needed and it is important that the therapist talk to the child to reassure and accustom the child to her. (This is especially the case with a preschool child, who requires more verbal communication in order to understand and become familiar with a stranger's use of language.) However, too frequent verbalization can be intrusive; it does not allow the child time to think and relax in silence. On the other hand, even with a totally silent child like Helen, if the therapist says nothing, this may increase the child's anxiety and sense of strangeness in the playroom.

The therapist also employed language to reassure Helen by talking through all her own movements in order not to startle her further. For example, the therapist talked about shutting the door, going to sit on her seat, where she would stay (and would have talked about the video or tape recorder had it seemed appropriate to use this with Helen). The therapist also tried to use language that would be readily understood by a six-year-old, using simple sentence constructions such as "You want to go and you want to stay", as well as simple vocabulary. Since the therapist had not heard Helen speak and Helen had not indicated that she understood what the therapist was saying, it was necessary to keep her spoken language at a basic level, roughly comparable to a three- to four-year-old's language comprehension. A further reason for keeping language simple is that an anxious child is unable to process complex information easily; anxiety will suppress higher level cognitive functioning. In addition, words with emotional impact will usually have the greatest effect if they are used simply and not embedded in complex sentence structures.

In creating a trusting relationship with her, the therapist also needed to consider Helen's use of personal space. The therapist attempted to respect this by remaining quite still and by not meeting Helen's glance when she noticed Helen looking at her. In general, in working with abused and frightened children, great care needs to be taken to respect a child's personal space. This includes being careful of the way in which one looks at the child. The therapist herself may experience a sense of intrusion and discomfort similar to that of a child if the child in the initial stages of therapy engages, as sometimes happens, in a lengthy scrutiny of the therapist's face. (This appraising look on the part of the child can be used to help the child therapeutically: "You are looking closely at my face" or "You wonder what I'm like" or simply by allowing the child to look without meeting her gaze.)

The therapist also reduced Helen's distrust by ensuring that Helen had the freedom to decide whether to remain in the playroom for the entire hour. If her anxiety became too great, Helen could choose to go back to her classroom. At the same time, the therapist built into her comments to Helen that it was not usual to end the session early, and that she expected Helen to continue to come to the playroom for further sessions. The therapist's expectation of Helen's ability to adapt to the therapeutic situation, in spite of and while recognizing her intense initial fear, was a critical dimension of the development of a trusting relationship between Helen and the therapist (see also Allen, 1942). The therapist's attitude was one of hope for Helen as well as a trust in her own ability to help foster healthy development in Helen. (This attitude will be discussed further in the general discussion at the end of this chapter.)

In these initial sessions with Helen, no mention was made directly by the therapist of the limits on Helen's behaviour in the playroom, for example that Helen was not allowed to hurt the therapist or herself or the room. Although it is sometimes necessary with a few children to establish firmly at the beginning a limit concerning destructiveness, in Helen's case this would have been frightening and superfluous. (See chapter 7 on limits.) Helen's behaviour was so curtailed that none of these actions would have been possible for her. The limit of the therapy session ending when the child left the room (a limit discussed in chapter 3) was referred to only indirectly – that if Helen chose to, she could leave the room and come back for the next session – but again, would have seemed inappropriate to state as an absolute at this stage. Helen's case illustrates the way in which, as Allen suggests, "Valid limits grow from the situation and belong to it" (1942: 72); rather than needing to be rigidly stated and imposed at the beginning of play therapy.

At the same time that Helen found these initial sessions frightening and conflicting, the therapist also had emotions and attitudes towards Helen, and feelings about her own capacity and desire to help her. Helen appeared unattractive, distorted in her movements and without any ability to relate to the therapist. At times during the hour, while Helen stood immobilized by the door, the therapist questioned her own skill and Helen's potential for healthy growth. It was extremely hard to see Helen's anguish during each session and to know that the therapeutic situation was probably heightening this emotion. The therapist at times wished actively to intervene, either by terminating the session or by trying to direct Helen's actions, in order to alleviate Helen's distress. A further struggle for the therapist, because of Helen's prolonged silences and lack of communication, was to keep attention focused on her.

The underlying attitudes the therapist drew on most in the initial sessions to sustain her were patience (Taft, 1933, in fact, points out that 'therapy' derives from the root meaning 'to wait' or 'a servant'), faith in the method of therapy she practised and hope concerning Helen's potential for emotional growth. Although Helen's emotional suffering in her presence was great, the therapist was aware that Helen had actively decided to remain in the room each week. The therapist had also firmly committed herself to twelve sessions and knew that she could not withdraw from the sessions without feeling that she had failed Helen and herself, Helen's mother, and the school, in that order.

These general attitudes of the therapist are not only necessary to sustain and give overall meaning to the therapist in her work; they also convey to the child the therapist's general emotionalized attitudes, including body language and other cues, that are beyond the therapist's ability to control and communicate directly (as the following section illustrates). In Helen's case, she seemed hypervigilant of the therapist, while trying at the same time to ignore her, (a phenomenon noted by both the Tinbergens, 1983; Miller, 1948). The therapist was unusually aware of the fact that her attitudes were conveyed to Helen on many levels and not just in the behaviours that the therapist was consciously aware of and which were under her own control.

Finally, the theoretical framework Erikson uses to describe the establishment of trust between parents and their children seems to have relevance to the therapeutic relationship. (We will discuss this framework more fully in the next chapter.) Helen's extreme fright and mistrust of the therapist seemed to parallel a failure to develop an emotionally trusting relationship with her mother and perhaps with all other adults.

THE MIDDLE SESSIONS: THE STAGE OF FALSE INDEPENDENCE

The middle sessions of Helen's therapy can be subdivided, in retrospect, into four different stages: the stage of a relationship of false independence from the therapist; the stage of mutual sharing; the stage of symbolic play and, finally, the stage of self-controlled regression.

In this middle stage, Helen progressed into a stage of false independence from the therapist. (Ekstein, 1966, defines this as a "quasi-symbiotic" relationship with the therapist.) This relationship is one in which the child seems to act independently and forces the therapist into a dependent, imitative situation. The therapist becomes the child's mechanical reflection in that she must perform actions at the child's direction. For Helen, this shift began in her fourth session. The session began with Helen exploring the room and equipment again, but this time moving further from the door. She then abruptly unwound a long roll of paper which was nearby and stretched the paper across the entire length of the room. The therapist, remaining in her usual stationary position, remarked that Helen had found something she wanted to do. Helen disregarded the therapist's comment. With her head down, she grabbed a crayon from the shelf and placed herself at one end of the paper. Without glancing up, she commanded the therapist to go to the other end of the roll and draw **exactly** what she was drawing. Helen's words were perfunctory, consisting of short, barking commands: "Go there." "Do this." "No, like this."

The therapist followed Helen's commands, commenting briefly on her own actions to reassure her: "I'll get a crayon from the box", as she rose from her chair; "You want me to do what you do"; and "Mine isn't just the same as yours." The therapist was aware that Helen was testing her and that she needed to take great care not to frighten Helen by her actions or remarks. The therapist drew exactly what Helen did – very easily imitated curved lines – making occasional brief remarks about what they were both doing. After about fifteen minutes of this activity, the therapist expressed restiveness, saying it was hard to do just what Helen wanted her to do. Helen, without looking at the therapist, said "You have to", with great emphasis. The therapist replied that it was important to Helen for the therapist to do what Helen told her to do. And added that it was hard to do just what she was told for a long time. Helen said angrily "Don't talk" and continued silently to draw lines, taking long pauses between actions. The therapist, too, continued to follow her lead in silence until the end of the hour, when, as usual, the therapist reminded Helen that the clock would be at "eleven o'clock" soon and it would be time to leave.

In the next two sessions, Helen's exploratory, fragmented actions were no longer confined to the area around the door but covered the entire space of the room, including the area near the therapist's chair. Helen's exploration was interspersed with drawing on the paper roll, with the therapist and Helen always positioned at opposite ends of the paper. Gradually, Helen commanded the therapist to imitate her in coming closer and closer together, drawing lines that brought them both towards the middle of the roll of paper so that by the end of the sixth session they were drawing shoulder to shoulder, at the middle of the paper. Throughout these sessions, however, Helen did not want the therapist to talk, and she herself was silent except for issuing peremptory commands.

DISCUSSION OF THE STAGE OF FALSE INDEPENDENCE

This stage in the therapeutic process seems to be characteristic of a child who either has severe difficulty in establishing a trusting relationship with an adult or who is very young and frightened. As Ekstein remarks, the commands issued by such a child are reminiscent of "the way a tyrannical, small child might control the mother who must never be out of his sight and is used as an extension of the child". (1966: 69) One of the emotional meanings of this extreme behaviour for the child, then, is safety. Using Erikson's framework, the child can be viewed as not having built up a trusting relationship in which he is capable of distinguishing the outside world from his inside world. He cannot differentiate between himself and others because he is not able to trust those outside himself and therefore cannot trust his own actions either. By controlling the situation, the child can reduce both the outside and inside threats to his safety at the same time.

Helen's false independence from the therapist seems to be a distortion of the natural progression in a child's emotional development, with a pretended and hostile autonomy, rather than a healthy emotional progression to true autonomy. Helen, after forming a very rudimentary trust in the therapist, seemed to be moving on to Erikson's second stage of emotional development, that of autonomy versus shame and doubt. However, due to great difficulties in Helen's emotional development, her sense of mistrust in herself and in the therapist still dominated her relationship with the therapist. Helen made the therapist into her mechanical reflection and was unable at this point to progress fully into the next stage in their relationship.

Non-directive play therapy seems particularly suited to a child's need to work through this stage of false independence in his emotional development. In non-directive play therapy, as we have stated, the child takes the lead in directing his own behaviour. When Helen initiated the action with the roll of paper herself, it was readily apparent that she was moving on to a different stage of therapy. Helen, too, could see that she took the initiative in this new relationship and probably began to trust the therapist to help her at her own pace. The therapist knew that Helen was ready to have different responses made to her because it was Helen herself who initiated the action; the therapist, therefore, could acknowledge and quite easily respond appropriately to this new action. The therapist was confident, then, that she could help Helen to become aware consciously of this shift in her feelings. At the same time Helen's actions gave the therapist the opportunity to ready herself for new actions from Helen with, perhaps, different emotional contents.

As the therapy sessions unfolded, it was obvious that Helen had adopted her own unique symbolic means of conveying her feelings about herself and her relationship to the therapist, creatively using materials in the room for this purpose, rather than words. In fact, the therapist's and even her own language was so threatening to her that she commanded silence, after tolerating only a few remarks by the therapist on a feeling level. The paper roll, rather than language, was used to demonstrate the beginnings of trust which Helen felt in their relationship. Helen engaged the therapist in the shared action of drawing, but only when she could exercise complete control over the therapist's actions and words, thereby reducing the threat this change in the relationship posed for her. She was also able to indicate nonverbally that her feelings towards the therapist were changing by allowing herself and the therapist to reduce the physical space between them (she was still not able to tolerate face-to-face contact, however).

The therapist's comments, then, were only used briefly, but they served to mark both the change in the relationship and the emphasis placed by the therapist on Helen's feelings. It was important therapeutically for the therapist to hypothesize that Helen was placing her in a dependent position and that the therapist should use the feelings engendered in her by this role in a congruent way, at the same time realizing that Helen could not easily tolerate verbalization of these changes in feeling. The therapist, by acknowledging her feeling of restiveness and her difficulty in following Helen's directions was able to demonstrate to her how Helen herself might feel in emotionally similar situations. Helen's simple actions and words, and the therapist's replies, must have had both emotional impact and a variety of personal meanings for Helen, although the specific contents of these meanings would be known only to Helen herself, and not to the therapist.

The therapist, by permitting herself to be placed in a dependent role by Helen, was demonstrating clearly to Helen what their potential relationship might be. Role playing in non-directive play therapy allows the child to direct the adult, to make the adult in important respects into what he wants her to be. The environment is thus seen as permissive in unique and therapeutically important ways. It should be noted, however, that Helen's use of the therapist as her mechanical reflection indicates a disturbance in Helen's ability to role play (a subject which we considered more fully in chapter 2).

THE THIRD STAGE: INITIATIVE AND MUTUALITY

The third stage in Helen's therapy was marked by her beginning to play and to establish a relationship of mutuality with the therapist.

Following the session in which Helen and the therapist had drawn on the paper shoulder to shoulder, Helen drew briefly on the roll of paper and then walked over to the easel and painted several paintings in quick succession. These paintings were copies of the simple curved lines she had drawn on the roll of paper. After finishing the paintings, Helen left the easel and walked around the room close to the easel, looking at other toys and looking back at the easel. The therapist, sitting in her usual position, commented briefly and quietly on Helen's actions: "You're drawing again ... You're going to do something else now ... You're doing them the same ... You're being quick ... You're thinking about painting again." Any emotive comments were still judged to be highly threatening and as Helen was still silent, implying that she did not want to engage in conversation, the therapist kept her comments minimal.

Helen approached the easel again, took the paint pot and began cautiously to spill a bit of paint. With each few drops that she poured on the floor, Helen looked closely at the therapist. The manner in which she spilled the paint was, somehow, both 'accidental' and contrived. The therapist, while Helen was spilling the paint, remained in her seat and commented: "You want to see what I think when you're spilling the paint ... You can do things in the play-room ... You can't do that in other places." After several small spills, Helen noticeably relaxed physically. She gave fleeting smiles to herself and her body relaxed somewhat from its taut stance. As the session ended, Helen seemed able to walk out more easily.

The next session was entirely exploratory, with Helen walking around the room. But Helen's exploration this time was very different from her fragmented, stilted movements from toy to toy in the first sessions. The therapist commented more frequently on Helen's progress around the room, with remarks such as: "You're interested in the toy telephone ... You're wondering what's in there", trying gradually to introduce more feeling words on a non-threatening level. Helen responded by continuing her exploration of the room, and glancing at the therapist from time to time, especially when the therapist commented on what she was doing.

At the beginning of the next session, Helen came into the therapy room, announcing that her teacher had allowed the class to do foot painting, but she had been in trouble because she had made a mess all over the outside pavement and not just on the paper. Helen wondered aloud to herself whether she could do that in here, at the same time removing her shoes and socks. She took the paint pots from the easel one at a time and poured them all into a pool on the floor. Helen stepped repeatedly in the paint, and finding some pictures on a shelf nearby, threw them up into the air and let them land in the pool of paint on the floor. Helen then offered a picture to the therapist and told her to "throw the picture in the mess". All the time Helen was engaged in making the "mess", she was both self assured in her actions and interactions and very relaxed. Rather than her previous manner of gleeful naughtiness around adults, this time Helen was openly laughing with the therapist and looking directly into her eyes, while standing face to face, for long periods of time. There was a deep sense for both of them that they were enjoying doing it together, which the therapist reflected to Helen.

After finishing, Helen asked the therapist to help clean her feet. The therapist scrubbed Helen's feet in the basin, after Helen had climbed up onto the draining board in the kitchen area. Helen dried her feet and put on her shoes and socks, ready to go. She then turned to the therapist and asked with concern about who would clean the room. The therapist commented that Helen cared about the room and wanted it to be clean again. She also reassured Helen that she would clean the room after Helen left. Helen smiled and went out of the room happily.

Helen made a "mess" each time for the next three sessions, all of them following the same pattern. At times while tossing pictures in the air, she would look with interest at the picture and comment briefly on it to the therapist. She also played in short bursts with other toys in the room.

DISCUSSION OF HELEN'S THIRD STAGE IN THERAPY

After her rigid control of actions in the previous false independence stage in her therapy, Helen became able to initiate actions with a sense of purpose and with her own personal meaning. Helen allowed the therapist to make simple comments on her actions, and she progressed to being able to explore the room easily, while tolerating more statements on a feeling level by the therapist. She was then able to initiate an important and purposeful action, spilling paint. At the same time she seemed able to extend her interactions with the therapist by being able to look closely at the therapist while listening to her comments.

The therapist, when Helen began to spill paint, quickly decided that it seemed important therapeutically for Helen to experience a loosening of restrictions in play. She had inferred from her own feelings, which she had used congruently when she and Helen were drawing together, that tight rules governing actions had felt intolerably self-restrictive and frustrating to Helen. She decided in Helen's case to allow her to spill paint – as much paint as she had in the room, initially – rather than set a limitation on the amount of mess Helen was allowed to make. With another child, however, it might be more appropriate to set a tighter limit on spilling paint, depending upon whether the child was intending to make the room unuseable or whether the child was challenging the therapist to enforce a known limit. It is also important when a child knows a customary rule, such as Helen knowing that she must not spill paint at nursery school, that the therapist acknowledges the appropriateness of the child's known rule at the same time as stating that the therapeutic environment is more permissive. If the therapist fails to acknowledge the accuracy of the child's knowledge of basic rules, the whole rule system of the child and/or the child's belief in the trustworthiness of the therapist could be called into question. As one worried four year old boy, who had several times tried to figure out a seemingly totally permissive therapist's rule system, declared: "We don't **really** eat sand here, do we?"

Two sessions after first spilling the paint, Helen entered the room and started talking to the therapist in an open manner and at length about the footpainting which she had done at school. This conversation was in marked contrast to Helen's previous sessions which had been filled with long, protracted silences. The therapist, having heard only a few words from her, was not until that point familiar with either her language or her mental ability and to hear Helen speak as a normal six-year-old was fascinating as well as somewhat surprising and disconcerting. However, the therapist's interested reaction to Helen's conversation was a private and personal emotion, rather than a feeling to be used congruently and conveyed for therapeutic purposes to Helen herself. Helen seemed completely and matter-of-factly to accept her interactions with the therapist, without any trace of self-consciousness. Sometimes, as other therapists have described, the speed of change in a person seems very rapid, involving as it does "a salutatory change of personality ... In any form of therapy, patients, when they do change, tend to do so in readily identifiable steps ... A sudden insight leads often to radical and far-reaching changes ... because the central structure is changed – a new self-concept has developed." (Corsini, 1966: 25; see also Rogers, 1951; Axline, 1947)

When Helen spilled paint and then decided to throw pictures into the 'mess', the therapist had to decide on her limits; this time on whether to allow Helen to get paint on the pictures. Again, the therapist decided on permissiveness, resigning herself to cutting out magazine pictures and pasting them on to card to replace the damaged ones. Two feelings of minor importance entered for the therapist here: regret that she hadn't put the pictures away, since others using the room obviously valued them; and dismay over the amount of time that would be required of her to leave the room as she found it. These feelings, again, were private ones, to be dealt with by the therapist, rather than having therapeutic value for Helen, because her overriding need seemed to be to make a "mess".

Helen certainly showed by her action of sharing the pictures with the therapist and throwing them in the paint together that she was capable of and ready for a new level of relationship. The therapist was aware that her personal reactions to making a mess were much more muted than Helen's were. The therapist was concerned, while participating and reacting positively and warmly to Helen's smiles and laughter, that Helen would be deterred by her reservations. The therapist had resolved her negative feelings about Helen making a mess in the previous session, but had not been confronted then with being an active participant in the process. Again the therapist judged that her inhibitions against making a mess herself were personal feelings, rather than ones to share therapeutically with Helen. The therapist's constraint was due, she believed, to her adult status and years of training in adult responsibility for tidiness; nonetheless she was willing to try to shed some of her reserve. The therapist seemed to have responded positively enough for Helen to continue her wholehearted actions without feeling inhibited or guilty.

The therapist also was aware of and responded to Helen's rapid escalation in nonverbal communication appropriately. She was concerned that she might not always keep pace with Helen's changes and felt under pressure to adjust herself quickly to Helen's increased intimacy. She felt comfortable with Helen's more frequent eye contact, with Helen's removal of her shoes and socks, and only slightly uncomfortable with Helen's face-to-face interactions which occurred for long periods of time during the session. These were very direct and included extended eye contact and laughing and smiling full face at the therapist. The other very intimate interaction to which the therapist responded easily was washing Helen's feet. In all these interactions it was Helen's spontaneity and lack of unease that helped the therapist respond appropriately. Her only difficult personal emotion was that because of her maturity and training she was more knowledgeable than Helen could be of the profundity of Helen's rapid changes and the implications of therapeutic progress that they demonstrated. At times it was difficult to control her sense of excitement and wonder at Helen's quickly escalating intimacy.

Another significant change in Helen was seen in her concerns about the room being cleaned. This concern often occurs with a child who has had either too rigid or inconsistent standards imposed on him in the autonomy versus shame and doubt stage of emotional development. (We refer in chapter 6 to the links between messiness and sexual abuse, but this is an issue which in our view merits further exploration.) He changes in therapy and becomes able to risk making a mess in the therapy room. Instead of continuing to want to make the room messier, at some point the child wants to be reassured that his mess can be undone, by himself or by the therapist. Otherwise he feels threatened by the initiative he has taken and guilty about the irreversible damage he has done. Obviously, this has therapeutic implications – the therapist needs to limit the mess to what can be put right again. And often a child will use the cloths, towels, dustpan and brush provided in the therapy room at this stage.

As the therapist conveyed to Helen, Helen's concern over tidying the room shows that she felt a regard for the room, for something outside her own needs and actions. She felt a sense of belonging and a sense of caring for what she valued and used; the sense of mutuality was developing in her.

As discussed above, Helen made a mess on four occasions and the therapist did not enjoy the task of tidying up after each session. During the ongoing process of therapy, the therapist had no idea for how many sessions Helen would continue to make a mess. She had to resign herself to the cleaning task because the activity seemed so necessary to Helen, and had helped bring about such deep changes in their relationship. She sustained the hope that Helen would progress beyond this need to make a mess and move on to an activity that was less tiring and time-consuming.

THE FOURTH STAGE: SYMBOLIC PLAY

After four sessions of "making a mess", Helen moved on to another type of play. She began by playing quietly with several toys, such as the toy soldiers and the dolls house, each for a short period of time. She spent the time between playing with the toys exploring other toys and areas in the room, especially the area closer to the therapist which she had ignored before. Helen then began playing with two hand puppets near the therapist, one an elephant and the other a monkey. After trying them on several times and moving the puppets on her hands, Helen said that the monkey was the bad one and the elephant was the good one. The therapist commented that in Helen's family there was one that was called "bad" and another one that was called "good", too. Helen immediately looked away from the therapist and removed the puppets from her hands. She then went to play at the end of the room furthest away from the therapist, playing with one toy briefly, then another until the end of the session. The therapist quietly commented that Helen did not like what had been said. Near the end of the session the therapist commented that Helen didn't want to be near her, that she wanted to play over there by herself. Helen did not respond, but played with her back to the therapist for the remainder of the session and left the session silently.

During the next session Helen began by playing briefly with toys in several different parts of the room. Halfway through the session Helen again picked up the puppets and started putting them into empty cubicles in a row of shelves. She labelled the monkey the bad puppet and the elephant the good one. The bad monkey always had to be in a tree, very high up, by himself in the dark. The good elephant was down on the ground playing. Several times during the session Helen took the bad monkey down out of the dark to join the elephant, but the monkey always caused trouble and had to be shut away again.

The therapist, while Helen was playing with the puppets this time, tried to follow the action and feelings Helen attributed to the puppets. The comments the therapist made reflected and clarified the feelings and actions of the monkey in the play sequence; comments such as: "The monkey is all by himself. Maybe he feels lonely ... It's dark for the monkey ... The monkey sees the elephant playing and wants to play, too ... The monkey's naughty again; he keeps fighting with the elephant ... The monkey's in the dark alone again ... The monkey keeps trying over and over to play. He just can't get along."

DISCUSSION OF HELEN'S SYMBOLIC PLAY

Helen began these two sessions by trying out different toys throughout the room. She trusted the therapist more and could explore the toys and area in the room around the therapist as easily as she explored other areas in the room. Helen seemed to decide on the two puppets, after casually playing with other toys, as important to her emotionally. Unfortunately the therapist interpreted to Helen that the puppets represented Helen and her sister, rather than remaining with the symbol (the puppets) that Helen chose to use. Because Helen's puppets so obviously stood for Helen and her sister, the therapist mistakenly judged that Helen would easily see this, too. (As we shall illustrate in the next part of the chapter, sometimes the therapist mistakes her own viewpoint for the child's.) Helen was not able to use this insight of the therapist and felt threatened, possibly rejected and certainly rejecting of the therapist for unmasking the symbol. The therapist stayed with Helen's symbols in the next session and Helen was able to extend her play and the expression of some of her strong emotions.

It was painfully clear that Helen rejected the therapist's interpretation of her actions. The therapist acknowledged this rejection to Helen verbally and hoped that the progress of Helen's therapy would not be curtailed by the therapist's mistake although she feared that it might be. In the next session, when Helen picked up the puppets, the therapist felt that Helen was giving her another chance, and attempted to reflect and clarify the monkey's and the elephant's feelings, thoughts and actions, being careful to use only the symbols Helen used and not to extend the symbols beyond what Helen conveyed. Helen was able to enact a drama expressing her powerful and painful feelings as long as the therapist used Helen's chosen symbolic means to express these feelings, rather than the therapist's interpretations of Helen's reality.

THE FIFTH STAGE: SELF-CONTROLLED REGRESSION

The fifth and most dramatic stage of Helen's therapy was one of self-controlled regression. After her session of playing symbolically with the 'good' and 'bad' puppets, Helen began her next week's session by putting the puppets in their cubicles, then taking them out, feeding them, and then putting the 'bad' one away. While playing with them, Helen started using a doll's nursing bottle that she had earlier taken over to the shelves to use to feed the puppets. She started walking around the room, sucking from the bottle, and letting the bottle dangle from her mouth. Then Helen sat down on the floor in front of the therapist's chair and started rhythmically sucking the bottle. After a few minutes her breathing became noticeably deeper and her eyes became fixed. Then, in a remote voice unlike her usual speaking voice, she told the therapist to pick her up and hold her. As the therapist held Helen in her lap, Helen curled up into the foetal position and continued rhythmically to suck the doll's feeding bottle. Gradually, she moved her body closer to the therapist's, until she was being held in the therapist's arms, against the left side of the therapist's body. Helen remained in this position for several minutes, sucking at the bottle, with the heavy nasal breathing characteristic of young babies while feeding.

Again in a remote voice, Helen told the therapist to put her down on the floor. She then dropped the feeding bottle and crawled around the therapist's chair, looking up and smiling as she crawled. After crawling for a few minutes, Helen got up and told the therapist to chase her. She unsteadily toddled away, looking over her shoulder and laughing while the therapist 'chased' her. The therapist responded to Helen as a toddler, pretending to be hurrying after Helen, clapping her hands and laughing back at Helen when Helen turned half around and saying "I'm coming" while clapping her hands and laughing. After being chased for a few minutes, Helen spontaneously reverted back to her normal speaking voice, talking about the toys near her to the therapist. Helen spent the rest of the session quietly playing with the toys near the therapist.

DISCUSSION OF HELEN'S SELF-CONTROLLED REGRESSION

Helen seemed to have reached the point in her relationship with the therapist where she was able to trust her to help her relive a normal sequence of emotional development. Helen seemed to 'live through' or experience earlier developmental stages which, from the information on her background, she had originally experienced in a distorted way (for example, the mother saying that

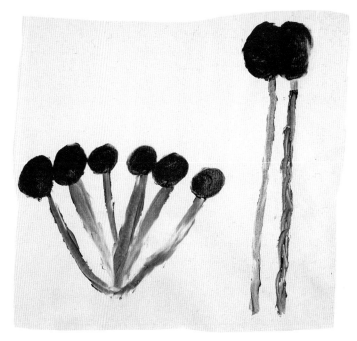

Plate 1

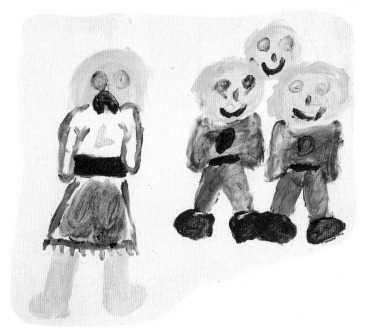

Plate 2

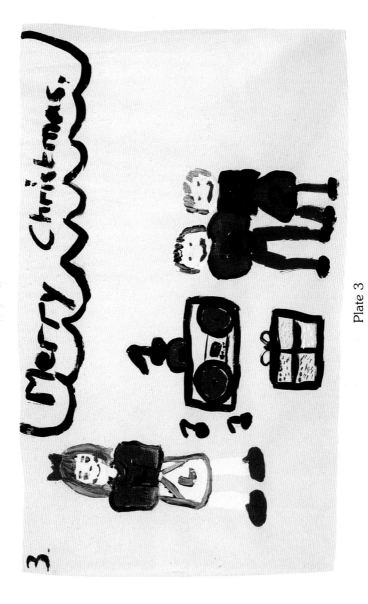

Plate 3

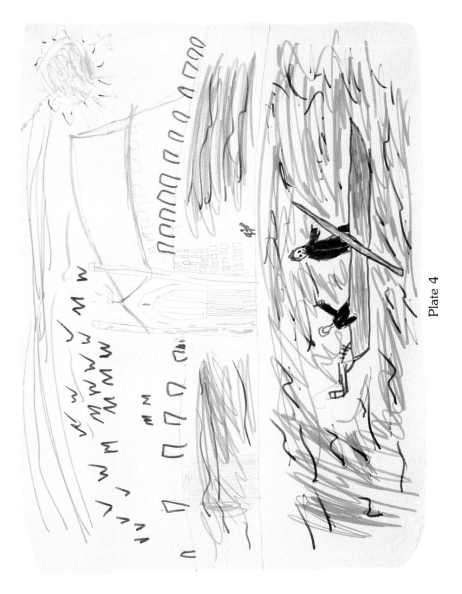

Plate 4

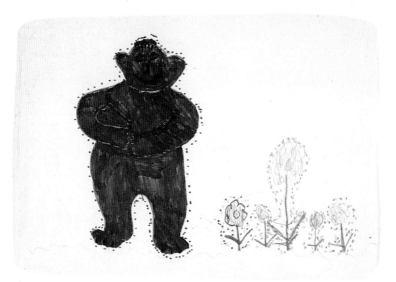

Plate 5

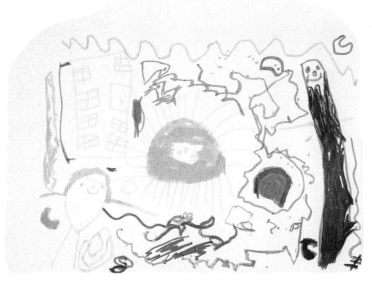

Plate 6

Helen as a baby "went rigid in my arms when I held her"). She appeared to pass through these stages at a vastly accelerated pace; at the same time she also seemed to 'live through' these stages. She did not simply role play or **pretend** to become a newborn, an older, crawling baby and then a toddler. The therapist had the uncanny feeling that Helen **had become** that age. She had the characteristic motor development, for instance, of each of the three stages she lived through. Helen was not a six-year-old child imitating a baby feeding, crawling or toddling, which looks exaggerated and inexact. Rather, Helen's motor behaviours were more or less identical in character to what one would actually observe in a child at each of these stages. (It would, however, be very difficult, if not impossible, for a six-year-old consciously to imitate the motor behaviour of a baby with this degree of accuracy.) Helen also exhibited the changing quality of relationship between a newborn, older baby and toddler with her parent.

First Helen wanted to be held in the neonatal position while feeding contentedly, completely at one with the substitute 'mother'. Then she gained some autonomy and separation from the 'mother', maintaining closeness by smiling up at the 'mother' as she crawled in a circumscribed circle around the chair. And finally Helen became physically independent and shared her enjoyment of her independence from the 'mother' in one of the favourite games of the toddler, chasing.

The therapist's role in helping Helen to 'live through' her earlier emotional development re-emphasizes that the child, in a very profound sense, knows what he needs from therapy and his point of readiness for experiencing emotionally important events. Helen's 'living through' experience argues forcibly against intervention and manipulation of the child's responses by the therapist. By intervening, even in an unobtrusive way, Helen's reliving experience could have been thwarted. The therapist's role is to provide appropriate responses, as indicated by the child experiencing this state. With Helen the therapist did not so much 'trust her instincts' as bring into use her past experiences. The therapist also was anxious throughout the 'living through' experience that any slightly misjudged response from her might bring Helen out of the fragile conscious state she was experiencing, thus hindering her progress.

The therapist, while recognizing the uniqueness of the experience, felt also in awe of something she could only partially understand. Indeed, no existing theory of consciousness known to the authors can adequately explain how a child whose own emotional development was so damaging to her could still know what normal emotional development is like to experience.

THE FINAL STAGE: INNER ACCEPTANCE, NORMAL PLAY AND A SHIFT IN FAMILY DYNAMICS

In the next therapy session following her self-controlled regression to infancy, Helen was transformed physically. In all her earlier sessions she had always worn shorts and a T-shirt, even though both her mother and younger sister wore dresses. But this session Helen wore a pink, feminine dress and had changed her hairstyle to having her hair worn in a fluffy way around her face, instead of being pulled severely back. The therapist commented that Helen looked very different today, that she had a lovely dress on. Helen smiled at the therapist and went over to the full-length mirror, always ignored previously, and looked at herself admiringly. The therapist commented that Helen thought she looked very pretty and that Helen was pleased with herself. Helen turned easily and smiled "Yes", turned back and smiled again, easily, at her reflection. She then went to play with the dolls house and quietly, contentedly played until the end of the session.

During the following week the therapist wondered whether Helen was indicating that her therapy sessions were ending and planned to discuss this possibility with Helen's mother. Before the therapist was able to contact Helen's mother, the mother herself asked to talk with the therapist privately. She discussed her amazement and pleasure over Helen's improvement at home – Helen's ability to get along with everyone in the family, her contentment and the ease the mother now found in caring for her. At the same, she expressed extreme anxiety over her younger daughter's behaviour. She described with anguish her sudden problems with her younger daughter, who had begun having violent temper tantrums and sleepless nights, and suggested for the first time that perhaps the problems were due not to her children, but to herself. The therapist recomended family therapy, along with individual counselling for the mother. The mother seemed relieved, agreed to try it, and a referral was made.

Helen had three more sessions with the therapist. The sessions were remarkable only because Helen was able to play and talk in a relaxed easy manner, with speech and play patterns characteristic of an intelligent six-year-old child. The therapist introduced the idea in the first of these three sessions that maybe Helen was ready to stop coming to see her now. Helen did not respond and the therapist commented that Helen didn't know what to say about the idea. It was planned that Helen would be transferring to another school in a few weeks and leaving the present school (and therapy room). She came to the next session talking excitedly about her new school, where she had gone for a visit. The therapist again mentioned that Helen was excited to be going to somewhere new and that maybe she was ready to leave the playroom as well as her present school. Helen nodded matter-of-factly and the therapist commented that Helen seemed to have that idea settled in her mind now. Helen then turned to play with the toys and played for a long time with the (fairy tale) finger puppets, inventing a story about the three little pigs being together, away from the bad wolf, in a nice new, strong brick house. The therapist reflected the pigs' feeling as they left their old house, worried about what they would find and feeling all alone, of being frightened of the big bad wolf, but now safe and happy together in a new strong house. At the end of the story, the therapist said that next time, since Helen was soon going to her new school, would be their last session together. Again Helen nodded in agreement and asked if she could go back to her classroom early because she was finished for today. The therapist agreed, said Helen seemed to feel ready to leave and that she wanted to leave early today. Helen smiled briefly at the therapist and happily left the session.

The last session was again a brief one. Helen came in announcing that she was going to her new school tomorrow and wouldn't be at this school any more. The therapist commented that Helen was thinking a lot now about her new school. Helen nodded in agreement and the therapist said that she knew Helen was ready to leave, but that she would miss seeing Helen and had enjoyed being with her. The therapist then gave Helen her own set of three pigs and the wolf finger puppets, so that Helen could play with them at home and remember all the times she had come to the playroom. Perhaps sometime she'd visit again. Helen was very pleased and asked if she could leave now to show them to her teacher and the children. Helen said she was going to tell them that she could keep them and bring them home to show her mum and sister. The therapist and Helen said goodbye, smiled and Helen happily ran back to her classroom with the present.

DISCUSSION OF HELEN'S FINAL SESSIONS

Helen's progression and readiness to end her therapy sessions were evident in every aspect of her life: she had changed physically as well as emotionally; and she had changed both in her therapy sessions and at home. The school had also noticed improvements. Because Helen had changed, her family's dynamics also changed (Satir, 1967). Helen no longer embodied all the family's dysfunction in her role as the 'identified patient'; her sister now was filling Helen's role. The family seemed to be attempting to regain its homeostasis which had been disrupted when Helen improved. But for the first time the mother could face her own responsibility for her children's problems and seek help herself. This shift in attitude was possibly because the mother, in seeing Helen's dramatic change, could overcome her own fear of inner change and have hope for herself and her family. Even though Helen's family was still experiencing turmoil and needed professional help, the therapist felt that Helen herself was ready to end her therapy sessions. The therapist based her judgement on the lengthy, normal play sequences and conversations Helen had engaged in with the therapist over several sessions. Helen's conversations and play drew on a wide range of current events and interests, for example, going to a new school. In addition, the therapist wished to exploit a natural break, Helen going to her new school, in order to effect an end to the sessions because this reason would be likely to seem sensible to Helen herself. The therapist then introduced the idea of ending the sessions and waited for Helen's response.

Helen at first made no response and then with the therapist's help easily incorporated the idea of leaving therapy into her move to a new school. She seemed to be able to accept the idea intellectually, as well as absorb the idea creatively on a symbolic play level, by inventing a story about the three little pigs. Helen also took control of the length of the last two therapy sessions by deciding to leave the therapy sessions early. The therapist reflected Helen's feeling that she was ready to finish. But the therapist also felt, since Helen was not acknowledging any negative feelings about leaving, that it was important for the therapist to use her own feelings of missing Helen and their time together therapeutically. By the therapist expressing genuine sadness and loss of their relationship, the child could have her own worth acknowledged, as well as seeing that it was a natural human emotion to experience loss, aloneness and sadness after a deep personal experience. The therapist was also aware that Helen's changes had been very rapid and that the family was still experiencing a crisis; therefore, the therapist gave Helen a concrete gift, finger puppets, to play out any later feelings Helen might experience, using the medium she had chosen herself.

SECTION TWO

GENERAL DISCUSSION OF THE PROCESS OF THERAPY

Helen's therapy sessions, because of the severity of her emotional problems and because the sessions easily divided themselves into distinct stages, serve to demonstrate quite dramatically what can be observed in a more muted form or at varied times in the process of therapy with many other children. In the following part of this chapter we shall discuss initial, middle and end sessions in more general terms and also from the varying perspectives of other children, as well as of Helen.

GENERAL DISCUSSION OF INITIAL SESSIONS

Helen's initial sessions were extreme in showing such acute fear, yet every child probably experiences some anxiety when he is brought to therapy sessions (Allen, 1942). Simply by being brought to therapy sessions, a unique situation for most children, an important message is conveyed to a child. The message of the carer (or agency) arranging therapeutic intervention is often that the therapist is seen as a saviour, and sometimes as the child's only hope for the future. But to the child, on the other hand, the therapist can be seen as a danger, because the therapist may be presented as someone who will 'fix' the child. The therapist can be seen by the child as an outside force, with the power to change him against his will (Allen, 1942). Even if the therapist's role is initially regarded by the child as more benevolent, the child will most likely still remain fearful of the unknown – the room, the therapist, and the relationship.

It can be expected, then, that a child will show some degree of diffuse anxiety in the initial sessions. It is important for a child to have the reassurance of a familiar and trusted adult waiting for him during the session and ready for him when he finishes (perhaps, early) at least for the initial sessions, and until he has indicated a readiness to allow the adult to leave during his sessions. (See chapter 3 for a discussion of setting up therapy sessions with a reliable and trusted escort.)

It is also important for the therapist to recognize and be therapeutically sensitive to a child's initial uneasiness. Some children exhibit ritualized actions with one object, such as putting a peg in a pegboard over and over again; others seem rooted to the spot and talk but cannot move; yet other children look at their hands, search their pockets continually, or zip and unzip their jackets, which they leave on. Once a child **is** able to make the first moves to play with the materials in the room, his play initially seems to be determined more "by the nature of the toys rather than by the use which they could be to the child as a means of self-expression." (Miller, 1948: 312) For example, a child who has started to play with the playdough will make playdough shapes using the cutters, rather than using the playdough as food for all the animals. The therapist also has a limited role in the child's play initially, usually being "a mere onlooker" (Miller, 1948), rather than being a participant directed in play by the child. Both the toys and the therapist are treated as objects outside of the child and are not being used in roles and activities that have special significance to the child. And when the child initiates conversation, it is usually more generalized and objectified, rather than highly personalized.

An example of another child (and another therapist) highlights the individualized responses each child makes during his initial sessions:

Billy begins the experience with a deep feeling of anxiety. He moves nervously from one item to another. The feelings of diffused anxiety are reflected in his constant questioning, his inability to decide, his wish to be dependent on the therapist, and his desire to be told what to do and how to use the play materials. (Moustakas, 1959: 106)

While the initial sessions provide important information for the child about the therapist, the therapist also has immediate insights into the child's unique personality and coping mechanisms because:

The child usually will respond to this new situation in a manner characteristic of the problem for which help is sought. He may be fearful or aggressive, demanding or placating, silent or overactive, and so on. Whatever the response, the feelings awakened are now experienced in the relation with a therapist, who is thus brought at once into a highly significant connection with the child's turmoil. (Allen, 1942: 60)

While it can happen that the therapist and the child immediately step into the child's deep and innermost conflicts, it is more common that the initial sessions offer clues to these conflicts in a muted or indirect way. An older child unable to talk about his experience of abuse may build a model village with a large lorry crashing into a motorbike; a young child who is very frightened of being locked up and alone may pile an assortment of toys into the playhouse and build barriers to prevent anything from getting out; a deprived and neglected child may not want to leave when the therapy hour finishes. A child, then, can immediately convey clues to his emotional problems through the use of toys and/or his behaviour in relation to the therapist. The therapist's role is to follow the child's lead and reflect the child's feelings, using the medium designated by the child as appropriate.

It is especially important during the initial stages of therapy that the therapist is sensitive to the level of emotion the child indicates he can tolerate, as well as the symbolic means the child uses to convey it, because both the situation and the therapist are strange to the child and fear-inducing. Beginning therapists in particular, are usually more able to understand emotional expressions of the child which are mirrored in his play, rather than expressions of his conflict which are mirrored in his relationship to the therapist herself. This is because similarly to the child, it is also more difficult for adults to step outside themselves and objectively evaluate their emotional impact on other people, especially when they must do so at the same time as participating in an ongoing relationship.

By the therapist's sensitivity to primarily nonverbal information from the child, the therapist can help the child overcome his initial difficulties, those stemming from risking engagement in the therapeutic process itself. The therapist is helping the child to structure the relationship, in the sense that she is attempting to establish with the child that they are dealing primarily with the child's emotions, how the child is feeling. The therapist establishes her role as helping the child to understand himself as he experiences emotions. By helping the child to recognize and come to terms with his anxiety over the room, over the therapist and over his expectations of therapy, the therapist is immediately fulfilling a therapeutic role. She is showing the child by doing therapy, rather than by verbal explanations. And the child, perhaps for the first time, is hopefully beginning to risk consciously examining his anxiety at his own pace and using the symbolic means he chooses to use, at the same time as having adult support while he does so. The therapeutic process immediately shows a child, then, that he is able both to live through and begin to understand his experience of anxiety.

The other crucial dimension of the initial sessions is that the therapist is attempting to establish trust between herself and the child. With a frightened and emotionally disturbed child such as Helen, the process of creating a trusting environment and relationship is often the most difficult and time-consuming stage in the therapeutic process (Erikson, 1977; Ekstein, 1966; Axline, 1947). Other children in therapy who are less emotionally disturbed than Helen often react to the first or middle stages of therapy in a somewhat different way, without a stage of extreme mistrust or of false independence. Often children with less severe problems do not have difficulty staying in the room with the therapist, talking to her and playing. However, it is often the case that (especially older) children choose to use toys by themselves, without asking (or wishing) for the therapist's participation. Some children build a miniature world and symbolically represent something of themselves in the way they create it (Lowenfeld, 1979). Others create action between playthings, such as between two soldiers fighting, with one soldier who is the hero. Yet other children make things on their own, such as making clay pots. One noticeable characteristic of the first sessions with some less emotionally disturbed children is that the therapist is an onlooker, rather than a participant in any action. The child seems to use this initial period not only as a period to explore possibilities for himself in the play materials, but also to remain at a distance from the therapist. The child can in this way evaluate the therapist's reactions to and comments on his playing, becoming more familiar with the therapist and the expectations which arise out of the situation, and more convinced of the therapist's trustworthiness before engaging her on a deeper level. In fact, the absence of an initial period of reserve in older children is noteworthy in itself, and should give rise to concern.

Sometimes the child may appear not to notice or be concerned about the therapist, but again this may be a means of reducing his anxiety. One therapist described an emotionally troubled child who seemed to be totally unaware of the therapist and completely self-absorbed, yet became very disrupted in her play patterns when a new therapist had to be introduced midway into her sessions (Miller, 1948): a practice to be avoided and which, it should be noted, should only be considered in very exceptional circumstances.

GENERAL DISCUSSION OF THE MIDDLE SESSIONS

In the middle sessions the child increasingly engages the therapist and increasingly explores his inner world with the therapist's help, either through symbolic play or through symbolic self-expression, such as painting. Sometimes the child's deepening levels of self-expression and change can seem very rapid, as in Helen's case. The therapist might have greater difficulty in opening herself up to such a rapid increase in intimacy than the child. As an adult the therapist will be more aware than a child could be that an increase in intimacy will make the link between two people much more powerful.

It should be noted that this increase in intimacy and, in particular, the kind of extended eye contact which Helen engaged in with the therapist, is different from the searching and exploratory eye contact children use to try to figure out 'who this new person is'. This exploratory eye contact, often used at the beginning of the therapeutic relationship and seen most directly in young children, usually makes the therapist feel uncomfortable. It is important to use this feeling of discomfort therapeutically, for the child's benefit, in two different ways. First, the therapist's sense of discomfort can be a signal for the therapist that the child is vigilantly checking her out and the therapist can use this signal to comment on the child needing to look at her a lot to see who she is. Or she may comment that the child doesn't know her very well yet. Or it might be more appropriate to convey these messages non-verbally, by offering her face openly to the child to scrutinize and not averting her face or eyes. Note that the therapist does not refer to the discomfort itself, which is a personal emotion for the therapist to deal with internally. Note, too, that the therapist's own sense of discomfort is important to recall when the therapist is looking at a child and the child looks uneasy and looks or turns away. It is likely that the child is experiencing this same level of discomfort from too intrusive eye contact by the therapist. Recalling her own feeling of discomfort, the therapist will then be more able to modify her eye contact to suit the child's needs.

Besides eye contact, other nonverbal communications such as touching, and spatial distance from the child (as well as verbal communication), can be adapted to the child's signals more easily when the therapist understands their effects on herself and on her own feelings of increased intimacy.

Although Helen's changes during the middle sessions were rapid, other children may fall at the opposite extreme. Instead of rapid leaps, the therapist may feel that the child is going at a snail's pace. Conducting non-directive therapy at the child's pace may mean that the therapist has to wait very patiently during the middle sessions for small shifts to occur, or plays the same games or role plays repeatedly session after session. (Note that since the therapist does not direct therapy, the resistance felt is inside the child himself and not against the therapist.) The structuring of sessions into blocks, with a review after each block, takes into account slowly progressing children. Both the therapist and the child have endpoints in mind at the outset; the child may not wish to or be able to change rapidly. After an initial group of sessions, the therapist can evaluate progress in the child's home and school environment to assess whether more rapid or important changes have occurred elsewhere if not in the session itself, and the therapist and child can also decide whether further sessions are suitable.

In general during the middle sessions the child works his way towards deeper levels of emotional expression, using his unique means of self-expression, such as puppets, role plays, painting, and even self-controlled regression, as Helen did. And the therapist uses a variety of therapeutic skills with different children during the middle sessions, and as a result greatly increases her understanding of each child. Every therapist, however, needs to be able to accept that she will never know everything about the child she works with. In fact, paradoxically, it can seem that she understands **less** of the child as therapy progresses. This is because with therapeutic progress the child becomes less trapped in his pervasive emotional conflicts, which are manifested in almost all his behaviour in early sessions, as Helen's were, and becomes more sure of his own direction and therefore more spontaneous and creative in his responses. Of course, this is also exactly what can make therapy so stimulating for the therapist. Each session does indeed bring a new child into the room and demands a new relationship to him. It means that the therapist must be continually and actively searching for new meanings and new responses to each child in every session.

GENERAL DISCUSSION OF ENDING THERAPY

In Helen's case discussed above, it was relatively straightforward for the therapist to decide that Helen seemed ready to end therapy sessions (or to "graduate" as Allen, 1942, describes it). Some indications of readiness to end are: first, a child playing and relating to the therapist at the general level appropriate for her age; the child's changed behaviour at school and at home; and the child himself indicating that therapy sessions are becoming less important and that outside concerns are becoming more dominant.

For example, a three-year-old girl demonstrated the new importance of her adoptive parents in her life. This was apparent in her drawing pictures to bring home to both of them during the session and by talking about what each of them liked. And in Helen's case she shortened the length of the therapy session itself in order to be more involved in her normal school environment.

For another child, Mary, who was six years old, however, the therapist introduced the idea of therapy sessions ending near the end of ten sessions. There were indications, such as normal play and improved behaviour at home, that Mary could be ready to end her sessions. But Mary rejected the idea strongly. She interrupted the therapist and loudly talked about something else, masking the therapist's words. She also had difficulty leaving at the end of the session, as she had during her initial sessions and exhibited strong aggressive feelings towards the therapist when the therapist mentioned that the hour would end soon. The therapist acknowledged Mary's feelings and decided to address the issue during the following session if Mary allowed her to. The therapist, in trying to make a decision on the number of further sessions, in the meantime had a conversation with Mary's foster parents. They indicated that her behaviour at home during the week had been aggressive towards her younger sister, as it had been before therapy began. At their next session, the therapist said that Mary hadn't liked the idea of leaving and hadn't wanted to talk about it last time. Mary nodded and the therapist suggested that maybe it was too soon, that she needed lots of sessions, ten more, until the long summer holiday (again structuring the ending at a future date and not leaving it open-ended). Mary very seriously replied that she **needed** to come and the therapist readily acknowledged her strong need. (Note that this need is different in quality and intensity to the child reliving his earlier difficulties at leaving to make certain of his health and independence.) Mary was able during the following sessions to shift to a deeper level of playing out more complex, damaging emotions, using the therapist in the role of her mother.

In some cases a reversal takes place and the child takes the ending out of the therapist's control, making the decision himself. Edward, a twelve-year-old referred for delinquent behaviour and aggression at home following his father's disappearance, attended therapy sessions in his oldest clothes. The therapist and Edward had contracted ten sessions together. Edward explored many feelings and used the sessions in a fruitful way. He also commented on his own changes in behaviour outside the sessions. At the eighth session the therapist reminded Edward that they had only two sessions left. The therapist also mentioned that the time had seemed to go by very quickly and that she herself would find it difficult to say "goodbye" to Edward.

For the ninth session Edward had transformed his appearance and dressed in his best clothes. The therapist was taken aback by his physical change. She acknowledged Edward's "smart" appearance and yet the therapist felt at the same time that she was floundering to understand its meaning to Edward. During the session Edward began to complain about all the toys in the room while he was playing with one of his favourite toys, a pop gun. Edward said that they were "baby" toys, not nearly as good as real ones like bikes and football. The therapist reflected these feelings, saying that soon Edward wouldn't be playing with these "baby" toys, but would be playing with toys for older boys. Edward then said he couldn't decide what to play. After the therapist commented that nothing looked good to play with, Edward said he'd play something the therapist liked to play. At the end of the session Edward announced to the therapist that this was his last session, not next week. The therapist, recovering from her surprise, said that Edward wanted to decide when to stop, that he didn't want the therapist to tell him. The therapist added that it was up to Edward, that she would be there next week in any case. The therapist then said that she would say goodbye to Edward now, and how much she had liked being with him. Although the therapist returned the following week, Edward did not. It was the therapist in this case, rather than Edward, who had more difficulty accepting that the ninth and not the planned tenth session had been their final one.

Both Helen and Edward, it should be noted, signalled a dramatic internal change by a very noticeable change in their physical appearance. In general the therapist needs to acknowledge this change to the child himself as well as keeping in mind the likely internal changes the child is signalling to the therapist, to himself and to his environment. The child (or adult in therapy) often 'tries out' changes in the therapy room that he is wanting to make, because he is unsure of how they will feel to himself or how his environment will react to them. By trying out these changes first in the therapy session, the child can test out these changes in a safe and permissive environment, see an adult notice and accept the change, and then risk himself in his wider environment.

In general, mental health is difficult to define, except in relative terms. Especially with children who have difficult lives, some basic conflicts will usually seem to go unresolved. The advantages of the child feeling independent and able to deal with his own problems without therapeutic help, which termination of therapy clearly states to him, must be weighed against how important the child's problems still seem to himself, his carers and his school. The therapist, while the appropriate one to make the decision about ending, must try to understand the child's viewpoint and as far as possible make the decision a joint one (Ross, 1959).

In summary, the therapist must decide when progressive development is again spontaneously under way in a child and seems likely to be sustained. The therapist, according to A. Freud, (quoted in Ross, 1959) need not take the child in therapy further along (or "deeper") than all children are at that point. In fact, the therapist cannot safeguard the child against future dangers and must be willing to "let him take a chance". All adults in helping relationships with children (including parents) find it difficult to accept that it is impossible to be certain of safeguarding the child against future dangers and crises, which inevitably are part of living itself.

It is important that the therapist discuss the child's ending with the carers. Not only will the child's progress at home and school be important information for the therapist to use in deciding about ending the sessions, the therapist also needs to give the parents/carers the opportunity to express their feelings (say, that parents worry that they do not feel capable without outside help) and to explain, where appropriate, that sometimes a child temporarily tests out his new gains and makes uneven progress or has old difficulties reappear as the sessions come to an end.

This testing out is because both interruptions and endings can seem to a child like a rejection of himself. Unlike Helen's sessions, a natural break, such as the sickness of the child or the therapist, or the child's or therapist's holidays, often arises to interrupt the child's therapy sessions at some point. Interruptions, as well as the therapist's time limit on sessions discussed in the setting up of the sessions, are preparations for the child's acceptance (and the therapist's) of the short-term nature of this kind of therapeutic work.

With both interruptions and the final sessions, a child should always be given adequate time to prepare for the event, and have available the therapist's help in handling the feelings which arise. The therapist should always briefly give the reason for an interruption to the child at least two sessions prior to the break, yet the therapist should be aware that even with an explanation, the reason can seem arbitrary and rejecting to the child. The child also needs to know, and usually needs it repeated, when the sessions will begin again. There are different ways to make this concrete for the child, including writing it down on a piece of paper for the child, or marking it in the therapist's diary. And sometimes a postcard (posted **before** a week's holiday) can reassure a child that he hasn't been rejected or forgotten (Ross, 1959). But sometimes illness, either the child's or the therapist's, can be sudden and unexpected. Often, again, the therapist can mitigate the child's feeling of being let down by telephoning or sending a postcard, reminding the child of the next date.

In any case, regardless of whether preparation for an interruption has been achieved or not, the therapist needs to recall the interruption with the child in the first resumed session. If the therapist is congruent in expressing her own feelings, it often helps the child to express and clarify his feelings. In the permissive environment of the playroom, the child is often able to express anger at the therapist for the interruption, either through symbolic play verbally, or nonverbally. The therapist needs to be alert to these feelings, as well as her own probable feeling of guilt, and take care neither to minimize nor to project her own negative feeling on to the child.

In the final stage of therapy, the child often needs several sessions to come to terms with his mixed feelings about ending the therapy sessions. Certainly for many troubled children, ending therapy sessions is emotionally linked to ending other significant relationships, say to his natural parent(s) leaving him. The child usually has negative feelings, such as sadness, jealousy of other children using his time and room, and regret, wishing he could start at the beginning all over again. Sometimes, in fact, a child relives his former difficulties in the therapy session or at home in order to test out for himself, the therapist and his carers that his problems are now manageable. It is also important, however, for the therapist to realize that the child leaving therapy may have positive feelings. Some of these are that it confirms that he no longer has serious problems, that he's glad it's over, that he'll have more time to do other things.

The therapist needs to help the child clarify his complex and mixed feelings about leaving. Sometimes a tangible object, as in Helen's case, is the most appropriate reminder that the therapist is still thinking of the child and believes the child can work out his problems with his carers and without her help. In other cases the child himself develops a creative solution to leaving: he may bring the therapist a small gift; or he may spend the time looking though his paintings, deciding which ones to have the therapist keep and which ones to bring home himself. Whatever the solution, it is important that the child has concrete actions or objects which clearly mark the end for him. As the wild fox who was tamed by the Little Prince said,

"... One must observe the proper rites ..."
"What is a rite?" asked the little prince.
"Those ... are actions too often neglected," said the fox. "They are what makes one day different from other days, one hour from other hours ..." (de Saint Exupéry, 1943: 84)

The end of therapy, which has been an experience in which certain rituals, such as the same hour in the day, have already been built in for the child, needs to be marked in the child's mind as largely positive, though tinged with sadness and regret, and an event that he can remember. The therapist also needs to be aware of her own feelings throughout the final stage of therapy, and use these feelings to help and understand the child therapeutically. Sometimes the therapist has strong feelings and has difficulty handling her own reactions. If a child's leaving (or any other events in therapy sessions) coincides with serious personal problems, say her own child being seriously ill, the therapist might magnify or distort the child's feelings inadvertently.

Another difficult and disabling emotion for the therapist concerning ending can be guilt. Other constraints, such as the demands of work, lack of financing, changing jobs and moving, or the child's move, may abruptly terminate the sessions. These problems may lead to the therapist not being able to handle her own feelings adequately, and she may therefore be unable to use her feelings therapeutically for the child's benefit.

At other times, the therapist will have to admit her own personal limitations. Perhaps she cannot reach the child therapeutically or is irritated or threatened by his behaviour. (Hopefully, this will be rare. Child therapists do need to have to have a genuine liking for and pleasure in being with most children.) Or perhaps, having tested out the method under supervision, a student decides that non-directive play therapy is not a compatible way of working with children.

In addition the therapist, in assessing her limitations, must also be realistic about her long-term importance to the child. While it is necessary to be scrupulous in keeping appointments, preparing a child for interruptions or endings, and giving the child her whole attention and skill for an hour a week, the therapist should not exaggerate her own importance. Even though the therapeutic relationship is unique, the therapist should not undertake therapeutic work where she is the child's total emotional support. The child needs other people in his daily environment to derive emotional support from, and will increasingly do this as his emotional development becomes healthier. Provided the therapist prepares the child adequately for interruptions and endings, the child will be more able to keep his relationship with the therapist in its proper perspective.

The therapist needs to keep her own perspective on her therapeutic relationship with the child when ending. She attempts to use her own feelings to help the child acknowledge feelings he cannot face, or like Helen, is not yet experiencing when leaving. But the therapist because she is an adult, with a wider and deeper understanding of life experiences than a child, is sometimes more deeply moved and sees greater significance in an experience than the child does. The therapist, more than a child, would recognize the finality of the last therapy sessions and their uniqueness in both their lives. Yet the therapist must be careful not to impose this adult view on to the child.

The last session, even more often than other sessions, is significant on many different levels. The child might attempt to accelerate working through his feelings, perhaps engaging in frantic, disorganized play in the sand box or, at the opposite extreme, may become passive and unable to initiate any activity himself. Every therapist at times needs reminding towards the end of therapy sessions with a particular child that:

Activity (by the therapist) must not turn into dominance, passivity must not imply disinterest, and neither is right for every (child) or any (child) all the time. The skilled therapist must adapt his behaviour to the specific needs of the child at any particular phase of treatment. (Ross, 1959: 93)

This demand is balanced by the relationship that has now developed between the therapist and the child: the therapist has much more insight into this child's recurring conflicts and new hopes. For the final sessions the therapist needs to be especially aware of the child's immediate and conflicting feelings and be able to reflect these feelings back to him. The therapist may also need to make the ending less final or less abrupt, if the child seems to need additional reassurance. Almost all children need to hear that the therapist likes them and has valued their time together (Ross, 1959). Some children may also need to know that the therapist will try to see them if they have problems and need help again. Other children need a more gradual withdrawal, seeing the therapist once a month, say, for a few months. Yet other children may need to keep some indirect contact with the therapist, perhaps calling on the telephone and talking at an appointed time with the therapist for a few weeks. With younger children, as with Helen, a small but meaningful gift from the therapist might be appreciated and valued. In yet other cases, it seems appropriate to send the child a postcard from time to time, or to send a card at a significant time in the child's life, for example on his birthday.

Throughout the process of therapy, and especially when the child is ending the sessions, the therapist must sustain her faith in the child. She must have faith, too, that the process of integration of past experiences and the creative use of current experiences which therapy helped the child set in motion and value in himself will be a firm enough base to nourish his further emotional development.

Having considered the general process of therapy, and illustrated this process by a discussion of the case material of Helen, we turn in the next chapter to a consideration of the particular themes which may emerge in therapy with children at different stages of development.

5

Emotional Development and Play Therapy

S E C T I O N   O N E

EARLY EMOTIONAL DEVELOPMENT

We have referred to the development of trust in the previous chapter when we discussed a child's general therapeutic progress. In the initial sessions trust in the therapist or autonomy from the therapist can be dominant issues, as they were in Helen's case; later, initiative and mutuality emerged in Helen's play therapy sessions. This chapter will develop these stages in emotional development – trust, autonomy and initiative – in more detail, as well as going on to discuss the emotional development of middle childhood and adolescence. By using this sequence of emotional development we intend to clarify the manner in which specific themes may emerge in therapeutic work for children of different ages.

While in our opinion no sufficiently comprehensive and detailed theory of normal emotional development has as yet been formulated in psychology, we have attempted to set emotional development and play into the broader framework of mental development (see chapter 2) by arguing that the child develops mental schemas which incorporate motor, affective (emotional) and cognitive components. Erikson's stages of emotional development (1963; 1964; 1968), as presented in this chapter, are intended to supplement our framework of mental development by showing how a child progresses through these emotional stages in the life cycle and how this normal progression is reflected in therapeutic work with children.

Erikson's framework gives coherence and added meaning to our clinical experience with children in non-directive play therapy, as well as to our understanding of less troubled children. In particular, Erikson's stages in the life cycle organize the child's development of emotions based on social interactions, as well as on maturational processes within the child, into a general overview of normal emotional development. It is also a sufficiently complex framework to encompass common deviations from and arrests in normal emotional development.

However, at the same time as recognizing that Erikson's stages are useful descriptions of general emotional development in children, we do not accept his psychosexual mechanisms for this development nor his psychoanalytic assumptions of "the unconscious" (see chapter 2). Erikson's stages of emotional development also seem to be too nonspecific, as Stern (1985) demonstrates, for infant development. Stern argues that clinical categories, such as trust and autonomy, are not necessarily age-specific. Rather, he argues that at each phase of development certain age-specific behaviours reflect the child's current view of, say, his autonomy (for example, gaze behaviour at three to six months, gestures and vocal intonation at seven months, etc.) and are culturally as well as developmentally determined. Erikson acknowledges incipient forms of each stage of emotional development in earlier stages, but does not specify in behavioural detail, as Stern does for infancy, of what these incipient forms consist.

In spite of his lack of specificity, Erikson does provide us with a theory of emotional development of sufficient scope to encompass an increasingly specific knowledge of children's emotional development. Briefly, Erikson's first five stages in the life cycle are: trust versus mistrust during the first year; autonomy versus shame and doubt during the second and third years; initiative versus guilt during the fourth to sixth years; industry versus inferiority during the seventh to eleventh years; and identity versus role confusion during the twelfth year up to adulthood. As with any classification scheme of developmental changes, the ages are only general guides to developmental changes. Petersen notes that "chronological age does not appropriately index many developmental phenomena" (1988: 585); for example, the onset of puberty is used sometimes as the definite index of 'early adolescence', rather than age twelve.

We assume with Erikson, then, that there is a proper sequence of emotional development; that there can be false progressions in a child's emotional development; and that later stages of emotional development are prefigured in current stages (that is, that each stage exists in an incipient form prior to its emergence, Erikson, 1963). We also assume that each stage in development is a turning point, a crucial period for the child of "increased vulnerability and heightened potential". (Erikson, 1968: 96) Because of natural growth processes, the child necessarily develops a radical change in his perspective and in his interactions with persons and objects.

Another important component of Erikson's stages (1963; 1968) is that there are positive and negative potentials for each stage of development. The child must acquire a balance towards the positive, say trust, but at the same time must acquire some of the negative potential, say mistrust, in order to have healthy emotional development. Having achieved this positive balance within the first developmental stage, the child is not, however, completely protected from all new emotional conflicts and environmental changes concerning trust and mistrust. Rather, if the child's balance is towards the positive side of trust, he will be able to meet later emotional development with more ease and will be more likely to maintain this positive balance.

BASIC TRUST AND ITS RELATIONSHIP TO PLAY THERAPY

Erikson states that the re-establishment of basic trust, the first stage in normal emotional development, is the basic requirement for therapy with some kinds of emotional disorders, such as Helen's. It is clear from the background information about Helen that her emotional development began to be distorted in infancy. Because basic trust is the "cornerstone of a vital personality" (Erikson, 1968: 97) it develops in the baby an inner sense of his own trustworthiness simultaneously with a sense of the trustfulness of others outside himself.

Stern gives a more detailed explanation of this social development, incorporating current research findings in infant development. He demonstrates that it is likely that an infant during normal development is "predesigned to be selectively responsive to external social events" (1985: 10), thus never experiencing, as Erikson and other psychoanalytic writers assume, a period of undifferentiation between 'self' and 'other'. Rather, experimental evidence in infant development leads Stern to conclude that:

During the period from two to six months, infants consolidate the sense of a core self as a separate, cohesive, bounded, physical unit, with a sense of their own agency, affectivity, and continuity in time. There is no symbiotic-like phase. In fact, the subjective experiences of union with another can occur only after a sense of a core self and a core other exists. Union experiences are thus viewed as the successful result of actively organizing the experience of self-being-with-another, rather than as the product of a passive failure of the ability to differentiate self from other (Stern, 1985: 10).

This view of an infant, as actively constructing and experiencing his environment, including relations with other people, fits our framework of mental development presented earlier. The relationship between the inside and the outside worlds is being built up by the baby through remembered and anticipated sensations and images. These sensations and images, in order to be utilized in a normal way, must be "firmly correlated with outer predictable people and things". (Erikson, 1963: 247) As the baby's feeling of familiarity increases, and his needs are met and forms of comfort become familiar, his sense of the goodness of life develops, and a hope for and a trust in the future. Erikson states that the amount of trust developed by the baby is dependent upon the quality of the maternal (and we would add, paternal) relationship. This "quality combines sensitive care of the baby's individual needs" with the parent's own "firm sense of personal trustworthiness within the trusted framework of their culture's life style ... (Parents) must represent to the child a deep, an almost somatic conviction that there is a meaning to what they are doing". (Erikson, 1963: 249) Applied to non-directive play therapy, the development of trust is engendered in the child by the therapist's sensitivity to what the child needs, as well as the therapist's firm sense of her own trustworthiness as an adult, which combines with her belief in the child's ability to develop in an emotionally healthy way. A therapist, in an overall way, then, must convince children that "they can trust us to trust them and that they can thus trust themselves" (Erikson, 1968: 97).

However it would be misleading to assume that a total sense of basic trust is necessary for healthy development; an **exclusively** trusting attitude would lead to gullibility and great disappointments. At times, adults seem to mistakenly assume that a complete absence of mistrust in children – either of adults in general or therapists in particular – is a sign of healthy development in children (see chapter 4, 'The Third Stage: Initiative and Mutuality).

Erikson reminds us that the development of a preponderance of basic trust, whether it is developed in infancy or through the therapeutic process, is not a lasting achievement, "impervious to new inner conflicts and to changing conditions ... The personality is engaged with the hazards of existence continuously" (Erikson, 1950: 265). Wolff (1986), in summarizing the useful-ness of child therapy, concluded that while child therapy does not seem necessarily to prevent later emotional problems from developing, one should not underestimate its potential for relieving a child's and his parent's short-term suffering. We, along with Erikson, would not be quite as pessimistic as Wolff, because in our experience some children **do** seem to develop greater resilience to later conflicts and difficult circumstances. However, because of the complex-ity and uniqueness of individual life histories, the long-term effects of thera-peutic interventions are extremely difficult to validate in children (see chapter 3, 'Discussion of Helen's Symbolic Play).

THE DEVELOPMENT OF AUTONOMY

During the child's second and third years Erikson states that the main emotional focus of emotional development is the child's development of will. He defines will as "... the unbroken determination to exercise free choice as well as self-restraint in spite of the unavoidable experience of shame and doubt in infancy". (Erikson, 1964: 119) A child can have severe conflicts at this stage in emotional development if outer control by his carers is not "firmly reassuring". Because he is in the process of developing his will, his behaviour can be at one time demanding, wilful and stubborn and at other times very pliant to adult requests.

The child is in the process of learning a **mutual** limitation of wills. That is, the child is learning "to control wilfulness, to offer willingness and to exchange good will". (Erikson, 1964: 119) The parent or therapist must adjust to this new emotional growth in the child, to the child's increased individuality. Applied to therapeutic work with children, it is essential that the therapist will have thought through the necessity for the limits (rules) she imposes on the child at different stages in the therapeutic process. These limits have meaning for her, as well as being "firmly reassuring" for the child.

The child who is referred for therapy often has had his growing sense of autonomy, or 'will to be oneself' thwarted at this stage in his emotional development. This may occur as the result of care which has been too restraining, to the point of trying to destroy the child's will, or too inconsistent, with the carer failing to protect the child from choices and situations which are beyond his ability and thus fill him with overwhelming shame and doubt in himself, and a pervasive sense of worthlessness (Erikson, 1968). Adults in these cases have failed to understanding and apply reasonable expectations towards young children: sometimes parents become infuriated with young children for being 'naughty' when the child is simply ignorant of what is to be done, or what is dangerous, or is as yet unable to control his emotions (Laishley, 1983).

Adults, unable to take the child's point of view, may fail to see that the child's environment can remain the same, but because his abilities and skills have increased, the child suddenly has many more possibilities and choices within this same environment. In non-directive play therapy this adjustment is clearly seen; the environment within the playroom remains the same, but the child himself changes. The therapist, in turn, must not simply 'remain the same' in relation to the child, but must shift her own actions and responses in ways which are based on the child's cues, as more possibilities open up for the child.

Negative feelings of shame and doubt can predominate at this stage if a child is not allowed to make enough independent choices. Some children whose independence has been stifled take a stubborn control over small things in which adults permit the exercise of autonomy by, for example, insisting that their toys be arranged exactly and not touched by anyone else (Erikson calls this the childhood form of the adult's obsessive behaviour). A child can also stubbornly exercise control over body processes outside the control of his carers, such as his own eating, toilet habits or sleeping, and become unreasonable and defiant in these areas because he is unable to express his autonomy in a more healthy manner.

In non-directive play therapy sometimes the initial sessions are primarily focused on the mother's (or father's) fear of relinquishing control over her child for the session with the therapist and the feelings of panic and helplessness that simultaneously emerge in the child (and the mother or father). At other times, the child himself defiantly tries to control the therapist's actions in the initial sessions. The therapist can then reflect the child's feelings of anger, anxiety and control, while allowing him to direct her actions, as the therapist did to some extent with Helen.

A child who experienced difficulty in the stage of autonomy versus shame and doubt was Martin, who was four years old when he began play therapy sessions. He was the eldest son of a single mother who also had eighteen-month-old boy twins. Martin initially doubted his ability to choose anything for himself, regardless of how small the decision. He was desperate to have the therapist decide which activity, which colour paint, which chair to sit on, and so forth; otherwise, he became immobilized by indecision. This pervasive doubt in himself seems to have started, as his mother explained, when Martin was just "asked to do simple things for her, like mind the twins while she popped out to the shops".

Young children, then, who have had either foreign over-control or continual demands and choices beyond their capacity, as seen above in Martin, often react in one of two ways. They may develop a precocious conscience, to punish themselves for not making the right choices all the time, which leaves them unable to act; or they may develop destructiveness and anger turned outwards towards others because they themselves have not developed the proper inner balance of free choice and self-restraint.

In non-directive play therapy, as we have shown in the above example and in the extended example of Helen, a child can re-experience his feelings of over restraint, defiance or doubt in a more permissive environment. The therapist protects him from choices and situations which are beyond his ability by setting limits, helps him to feel a lack of outer restraint by engendering a permissive environment, and allows him to express doubt in himself and his abilities. By experiencing and becoming aware of these feelings the child is able to begin to develop an emotionally healthy sense of autonomy.

Another negative outcome at this stage in emotional development, and seen in children referred for play therapy, is related to care-giving which either involves an almost complete lack of criticism or blame (what Erikson calls "shaming") or involves a preponderance of this, which is directed at reducing the child's autonomy. With a total absence of criticism, a child is unable to judge what is involved in a mutual regulation of wills and what his own realistic capacities should be at a given age. Instead, he will not be ashamed of or doubting of anything that he does.

In order to experience and work through feelings of autonomy a child often places the therapist, as Helen did, in the role of the child. Role playing is a very non-threatening and spontaneous form of play for children when they have both the power to initiate and alter the role play to suit their emotional needs and the power to put themselves into the dominant role. Helen seemed to have a disturbance in her development of autonomy, as we illustrated, as well as in her development of basic trust. The therapist must attempt to help a child develop a preponderance of autonomy, but she must also be aware that the child also needs to develop a more minor sense that there are also some things to realistically feel ashamed of and doubtful in. One of the main ways to do this as stated above, is for the therapist to convey a general atmosphere of 'emotional hospitality' and permissiveness to the child at the same time as imposing certain therapeutic limits that are 'firmly reassuring' for the child.

INITIATIVE VERSUS GUILT

Role playing is even more characteristic of the next stage of emotional development, initiative versus guilt. In Helen's case, she entered this stage therapeutically when she ventured to spill paint on the floor. Helen was beginning through this action to demonstrate a sense of purpose, characteristic of this stage of emotional development. A child at the stage of initiative versus guilt has a surplus of energy which permits him to forget failures quickly and approach what seems desirable, as Helen did with foot painting. A child also has a developing sense of realism about his abilities and is able to define more appropriately what he can attain and what he can share with others. Erikson (1968) states that the child begins to look outside the home for relationships with other adults. As demonstrated in the relationship between Helen and the therapist, a symmetrical relationship is being developed between important adults, especially the parents, and the child in which there is an essential equality between adult and child. This equality is based on the essential equality of worth of the child, even though there are obvious inequalities due to the child's immaturity.

The child begins to imagine himself as an adult; he freely imagines himself in adult roles, playing roles which promise to fulfil his range of capacities (Erikson, 1963). Children in the middle stages of non-directive play therapy often seem to have their imaginations set free and play a variety of adult roles. A six-year-old boy who engaged in highly circumscribed play in his early sessions took the role of a pirate, cook, father, postman and racing car driver in one of his later sessions, as he wove a plot around all these imagined adult roles. A child also begins to have meaningful social obligations and responsibilities, as demonstrated by Helen in her recognition of the social obligation to keep the pavement clean and in her concern over tidying the room.

Many children in play therapy seem to have developed a deep sense of guilt, rather than a preponderance of initiative, during this stage of their development. They feel responsible and guilty for imagined crimes, due to their vastly increased imagination, but can at times be unable to separate their inner from their outer reality. The therapist must continuously attempt to separate out the child's inner and outer reality for herself during non-directive play therapy, in order to be able to have empathy and reflect the child's feelings appropriately.

Very occasionally the therapist must ask direct questions (say, if child protection issues are involved; see chapter 7), but most of the time she would make inferences based on her knowledge of child development and on specific knowledge of the particular child. When the therapist is fairly certain that she has correctly inferred that the child is confusing inner with outer reality, she may sometimes help the child to make this distinction, as illustrated in the following example: Harry, aged five, had frequently played with a toy aeroplane and, looking very upset, crashed it into the sand. These feelings were reflected by the therapist, who nevertheless remained ignorant of the way this play sequence fitted into Harry's life. When the therapist visited Harry's foster parents before going on holiday, the foster parents remarked that they hadn't known how to explain to Harry that his natural father was in prison, so they had told him that his father had gone away in an aeroplane. The therapist, after explaining to the foster parents that children often worry more when they sense that the real reason hasn't been given to them for a major event in their lives, also discussed with the foster parents the way in which they could tell Harry about his father's imprisonment, making it fit the emotional and mental capacity of a five-year-old. During the next session the therapist introduced Harry to her holiday plans. She was able to help Harry clarify his feelings about his father going away and Harry worrying about the therapist going away on an aeroplane. She also reassured Harry that aeroplanes don't often crash and that she'd send him a postcard while she was away.

Because children have increased initiative at this stage in their development and many actions become possible, children also have difficulty and need guidance concerning their own responsibilities. Sometimes a child in play therapy blames himself inordinately for an action, say tearing a painting, which is the joint responsibility of the child and the therapist, or is sometimes the responsibility primarily of the therapist. In these cases, the therapist reflects the child's feelings without minimizing them, as well as using her own feelings of responsibility as an adult congruently to help him arrive at a more realistic view of his own actions.

Children's guilt and confusion over their own responsibility for actions can be increased with certain kinds of child-rearing practices. A child's guilt and confusion may heighten if his parents demand too high a standard from him, for example when parents expect that their child will never tell a lie, well before the age at which a child is capable of making the subtle distinctions among social lies, fantasy and lying (Ekman, 1989). Or a child may become confused when his parents apply high standards to his behaviour, yet he realizes that his parents fail to live up to these standards themselves. When this happens, a child can have a deep hate in himself for exactly the discrepancies he sees in his parents' lives. Instead of promising himself that he will be like his mother or father in their adult roles, as children usually do at this stage of emotional development, he turns away from this part of both his parents and himself. Finally, a preponderance of guilt and confusion can also occur if a child, in cases of sexual, physical or emotional abuse, is blamed for actions that are the responsibility of adults, rather than children. (See chapter 6 for a fuller discussion of sexual abuse.)

EMOTIONAL DEVELOPMENT DURING MIDDLE CHILDHOOD

During middle childhood, from approximately seven through eleven, a child develops a sense of industry. Erikson's stage of industry versus inferiority parallels other theorists' recognition of a major change in a child's development at around seven years of age. Intellectual and emotional development change qualitatively (Flavell, 1985); this change has been recognized in many different cultural contexts, as well as in psychological theories such as psychoanalytic and Piagetian theories. These intellectual and emotional changes during middle childhood enable a child to become more competent and skilled in a wider social context outside his family.

In the earlier stage of initiative versus guilt, a child could imagine himself in many different adult roles. With the now increased mental and emotional maturity of middle childhood, a child can now be formally instructed to become a "worker and potential provider" (Erikson, 1968: 124). A child's "exuberant imagination [is] tamed and harnessed to the laws of impersonal things". (Erikson, 1977: 258) During middle childhood a child seems to enjoy some direction and "likes to be mildly but firmly coerced into the adventure of finding out that one can accomplish things which one would never have thought of by oneself ...'" (Erikson, 1968: 127) In all cultures this developmental change is recognized and children receive some systematic instruction. In our own post-industrial society, school is largely separate from the family and from the adult world, becoming something of a culture in itself with its own goals, limits, achievements and disappointments (Erikson, 1968). Children at this stage need to develop a sense of industry and feelings of competence. Erikson defines competence, as "the free exercise of dexterity and intelligence in the completion of tasks, unimpaired by infantile inferiority". (1964: 124)

Another vital development, along with a personal feeling of industry and competence, is the child's development of a wider social identity. Erikson assumes that middle childhood is a most decisive stage socially because "industry involves doing things beside and with others". (1968: 126) The child is able to form deeper friendships because in working and in playing together in organized games, such as marbles (Piaget, 1965), soccer or gymnastics to name only a few, the child can "discover similarities of age, sex, style and aspirations in each other". (Wolff, 1989: 155) Stephen, for example, an eleven-year-old boy who had been sexually abused and now lived with foster parents, talked in play therapy sessions about how much his friendships at school meant to him: "My mates can make me laugh and help me forget about all my troubles."

Children at this age, then, need friendships and organized activities with their peers. They also need positive identification with those who know things and know how to do things in the adult world (Erikson, 1963; 1968). James, a nine-year-old boy who lived with his mother after his parents' divorce, talked about how important being in his football team was to him during his play therapy sessions, where his coach "acts just like a real dad, not like a teacher at all".

A child is able in middle childhood to have firsthand experience of the division of labour by having a position in a group, whether at organized games or in school tasks. In his group position he can compare himself, his abilities and his competence with others and can then place himself in relation to his peers. Within the world of the school, he can win recognition for producing things and doing things which would go largely unrecognized in adult society. For example, Gerald, a boy of ten who had an overwhelming sense of inferiority to his intellectually able younger brother, was able during play therapy sessions to make individual clay plaques for each of his teachers. Gerald was able to persist in his work and re-do plaques he found unsatisfactory, while the therapist reflected his feelings of effort, frustration and satisfaction, as well as his anticipation of the teachers' recognition of his efforts.

Several kinds of emotional problems emerging in this stage of emotional development are often seen in children between the ages of approximately seven and eleven who are referred for play therapy. One problem is that a child does not develop an inner sense of enjoyment or satisfaction in work or an inner pride in doing things well. Instead he seems to base his standards only on the outward appearance of the object, another person or himself, and the recognition by others as being competent or superior. This conformity, or the overweening need to have others recognize all his achievements as worthwhile, rather than his social need being balanced by an individual and inner sense of satisfaction in his work, can hinder emotional development. It can hinder a child from engaging in personally satisfying individual pursuits or it can distort personally satisfying skills, and result in these activities losing their individual basis for satisfaction (Erikson, 1968).

One girl, Lucy, who was aged eight, was referred to play therapy sessions because of paralysing shyness and withdrawal from peers. She asked the therapist, after some initial sessions in which she was largely silent, to tell her what to do before engaging in any play activity, as well as seeking the therapist's approval after completing each play sequence or creative activity. The therapist, while complying with Lucy's request, also reflected Lucy's need to have the therapist tell her what to do in order to feel she was doing it right. The therapist, in addition, used her own feelings congruently to reflect to Lucy that it was difficult for the therapist to direct Lucy's activities constantly because she didn't know all the things Lucy was good at or all the things Lucy wanted to do in the room.

In other cases a child can be referred for play therapy because either his family or his teachers (or, rarely, he himself) set unrealistic standards which he cannot achieve. These unrealistic standards often are incorporated into the child's own expectations for himself. He then becomes frustrated and angry with himself for his failures, and unable to work because he feels hopeless about achieving these unrealistic goals. The child, therefore, continually fails even easy tasks because all tasks have lost their meaning and purpose for him. This hopelessness and resulting failure increasingly reinforces the child's initial sense of inferiority and can lead to feelings of despair (and even suicide, especially in adolescence).

An example of this is Jayne, age eleven, who was both very overweight and becoming physically mature. Her parents complained that all Jayne ever did was "sit in front of the telly and eat, day and night", and they were extremely worried that she would be expelled from her private school for disastrous test results. As Jayne explored her earlier childhood feelings during play therapy sessions, she increasingly remembered times when she felt "alive and happy" while playing with her older brothers and doing "dangerous things", like climbing trees and playing in streams. Now, Jayne commented, there was nothing she was allowed to do, since her brothers had become adults and moved away, except study hard and stay at home. And her parents kept telling her how important her "stupid school" was and how many "sacrifices" they were making to send her there. Jayne wished her parents could go to that school they were so "in love" with and find out how "stupid" it really was. Jayne and the therapist then moved into a role play in which the therapist had to go to school and was unable to do anything right, always feeling stupid and unpopular. Over the next several sessions Jayne worked through her feelings of anger, frustration, inferiority and passivity with the therapist in the role of the student and Jayne in the teacher's role.

A child can also feel inferior when he differs greatly from other children in appearance, race, age or family circumstances. He may either require himself to conform rigidly to his peer group or rebel against his peers and school situation. A child during middle childhood learns how people outside his family, in his school primarily, judge his personal attributes (Wolff, 1989). If his family feels inferior and/or if he himself has experiences which give him evidence of society's devaluing of one or more of his personal attributes, the child may develop a debilitating sense of inferiority. He may also feel angry and frustrated as he becomes old enough to recognize differential opportunities in society and realize that only by chance is he being denied what others have. This frustration often surfaces in play therapy with the phrase "It's not **fair!**"

An Afro-Caribbean girl of eight, Delores, was referred for play therapy sessions after being expelled from school for acting defiantly and aggressively towards a teacher. The children in her family were all on the child protection register because of her mother's previous criminal record. Delores somewhat surprised the (white) therapist during her initial session by demonstrating that she had great skill in playing the musical instruments in the room. After playing several complicated tunes on a recorder, Delores asked the therapist if she could play tunes, too. The therapist replied that she wasn't able to. Delores then said proudly "My mum can!" The therapist reflected her feeling that she felt proud that she and her mum could do something well that the therapist herself wasn't good at. Because the therapist was able in this instance to reflect Delores' and her mother's talents, and not just their record of failures, Delores seemed able to make immediate progress in her play therapy sessions.

In the above case racial prejudice in a predominantly white society and family circumstances seemed to lead Delores to feel inferior when judged by societal standards. In other cases, family life may not have prepared a child for school life, so that nothing he has learned to do well earlier within his family is important to his teacher or his peers. As Wolff states: "Competence can make up for social disadvantage, and social advantage or esteem can compensate for limited ability. When both are lacking, children are in serious danger." (1989: 157)

An example of this feeling of inferiority occurred with a ten-year-old girl, Rita, who was in foster care at the time of referral, but had been forced to assume many adult responsibilities while still with her natural family. Her earlier childhood largely consisted of childcare and household responsibilities, with no allowance for or materials provided for activities such as drawing, painting, cutting or glueing. After Rita began non-directive play therapy sessions and started to trust the therapist's responses to a range of play behaviours for younger children, Rita began to use the scissors provided in the playroom. She used them initially in a clumsy and uneasy manner, watching the therapist's reactions and listening intently to the therapist's comments about Rita not being sure about using the scissors. Rita persisted, in spite of her embarrassment at her incompetence, for short periods in the next several sessions, but often became angry and frustrated when she could not manage to cut more than simple lines with the scissors. The therapist reflected Rita's negative feelings, as well as commenting that Rita wanted to practise with the scissors and get better, but it was hard not to be able to cut what she wanted right away. The therapist also hypothesized to herself that because Rita had failed to develop competency using scissors at an appropriate earlier age, she probably found herself excluded and constricted in any school or home activity with her peers that involved cutting. By the therapist reflecting Rita's feelings about her lack of competence in the permissive environment of the play therapy room, Rita began to use the scissors to her own satisfaction, although still not very skilfully, and managed to cut out stars that she had drawn on tissue paper.

Children, then, need the time and opportunity to develop skills, both at home and at school. They also need to have relaxation from organized activities. Some children referred for non-directive play therapy seem unable to make use of private time to engage in solitary play, say drawing, building models or aimlessly kicking a football without any apparent goal. (This difficulty in children seems to mirror certain adults' inability to engage in daydreaming activity. See Walls, 1972.) James, age ten, was difficult to work with in play therapy sessions initially because he felt compelled to fill the whole hour with organized ball games, without any rest periods. As the sessions progressed James and the therapist were increasingly able to explore his great uneasiness with pauses and his restlessness when not engaged in strenuous physical activities.

Other children seem to need more time for instruction from parents or other adults in order to produce real-world achievements of value. One nine-year-old girl, Mary, while playing with different colours of playdough, often expressed her longing to do baking and cooking at home. She put great energy and creative skill into pretending to arrange delicious food into pleasing patterns, and then serving them to appreciative people. Her frustration over failing to achieve real results in baking paralleled other child care patterns Mary was experiencing, in which there seemed an inability on her parents' part to recognize age-appropriate skills and abilities. Mary was assumed to be too young to understand a wide range of life problems and experiences and felt excluded, ignored and frustrated in her efforts to use 'real' materials to achieve 'real' results, as well as in her efforts to understand real life problems her parents had. In Mary's case, both play therapy and her school environment helped her to offset her home limitations. She turned to school and extracurricular activities at school for age-appropriate tasks and more age-appropriate interactions with adults.

In the stage of industry versus inferiority, as at earlier stages, a child needs to develop a preponderance of a sense of industry without being 'unduly impaired' by a sense of inferiority. Yet it must be recognized that each child does need to develop a certain degree of inferiority. He must begin to recognize that his pattern of abilities and achievements are to some extent unlike every other child's, and he will necessarily be inferior in some skills or in relation to some other children, at the same time as being competent or superior in other ways.

Adults, too, whether teachers, parents or other workers with children, need a firm sense of industry themselves. Sometimes adults feel inferior to competencies they see in children and ridicule or minimize the child's achievements. Or adults who have jobs without satisfaction or social status (or no job) may set unrealistic goals for their children because of their own career frustrations. One unemployed father of a boy, Robert, age ten, told the therapist at their initial interview that Robert would be coming to see the therapist as a concession to his wife, that as far as the father was concerned, Robert was "the most perfect child anyone has ever had. He's able to do everything – get swimming medals, get As, and play championship chess. What more could any father ever want?" Yet Robert was being referred for bedwetting and severe nightmares. The therapist suggested to the father that perhaps Robert didn't feel the same way about himself as his father did. That in any case the play sessions would be Robert's time for himself and private, without the need to do anything he didn't want to or talk to anyone else about what he said or did. In saying this, the therapist intended to convey to the father that Robert needed his own private life, not just a public life dominated, perhaps, by his father.

The therapist, as well as the child's parents and teachers, needs to have developed her own sense of competence. She needs to feel a sense of satisfaction and pleasure in doing her own job well and not be greatly threatened or made to feel inferior by superior talents in the children, or the parents of children, she helps. If the therapist does not feel competent, she may fail to empathize with the child's point of view and ridicule, minimize, overly praise or ignore the child's own feelings about his skills.

One common mistake made during early non-directive work with children is for the therapist to praise achievements in order to enhance the child's self-esteem. (See chapter 7 for a further discussion.) Not only does this praise often restrict the child's later freedom to make mistakes and prevent him from learning his own feelings about his efforts, but often the therapist mistakenly identifies her own feelings as being similar to the child's feelings. Robert, age eight, described at referral as of low intellectual ability, surprised an in-experienced therapist by drawing complicated and architecturally correct buildings during their initial sessions together. She conveyed her surprise to him and her admiration for his skill, but Robert insisted that the buildings "could be lots better" and threw his drawings away in frustration. The therapist was unable to reflect Robert's feelings, and only able to reiterate to him that she "could never do as well" and that "they were wonderful". In her later supervision session, the therapist and the supervisor discussed how the beginning therapist's sense of inadequacy and feeling of inferiority and inexperience, as well as her desire to enhance Robert's self-esteem, had blocked her recognition of Robert's feelings.

Another common problem in children during middle childhood is that a child may be unable to develop his sense of industry because he has failed to resolve earlier emotional conflicts. A preponderance of mistrust, developed in the first stage of emotional development, may impair all of a child's relationships and make it impossible for him to extend his emotional life outside his insecure home life. He may find the threat of separation too anxiety-provoking, as may his carers, to enable him to participate in school life. Or he may have developed shame and doubt in himself, leading say, to excessive withdrawal from peer activities and friendships. Or inhibitions due to guilt may develop in him a need to conform absolutely to teacher and peer pressures, rather than risk any initiative and, therefore, the experience of guilt which might ensue from his actions if they proved wrong.

In non-directive play therapy the therapist attempts to help the child over-come these unresolved emotional conflicts from his earlier development as well as furthering his current emotional development. As stated earlier, the child's intellectual capabilities expand, as well as his emotional capacity and motor skills. The intellectual stage of concrete operations marks an important shift in a child's mental life. He has become able to view himself as a thinking person and has more objectivity towards himself, as well as more distance from his physical and social environment (Piaget, 1967; Harris, 1989). The child is now able to think through and trust his own observations and conclusions about physical properties of the world, as well as have a more objective view of another person's position and feelings. He can also compare this view to his own view. But unlike the intellectual stage of formal operations developed during adolescence, the child from seven to eleven years still needs concrete objects and concrete experiences to arrive at correct solutions.

An example is Margaret, an eight-year-old, who was sexually abused over an extended period of time as a young child. Because of her abuse she was very unclear about sexual roles within the family. In her play therapy sessions she seemed to realize that she was confused in this area, often switching erratically between roles and assigning disparate roles to the therapist as well. For instance, Margaret assigned the therapist the role of baby and then immediately stated that the therapist should have a boyfriend. The therapist attempted to show to Margaret that she would fill her assigned role of baby-with-boyfriend, but using her feelings congruently, also commented to Margaret that it was difficult for her to play this role because babies didn't have boyfriends really; they were too young for them. Margaret continued to assign roles to the therapist, which the therapist carried out under Margaret's instructions. Gradually Margaret's role playing began to incorporate the appropriate sex roles she was now experiencing in her foster home. Margaret, then, by assigning concrete roles to herself and to the therapist, was gradually able to compare her own view of sex roles with those of the therapist and her foster parents.

The above example illustrates how during middle childhood the symbolic play in non-directive play therapy sessions becomes more complex than when working with younger children. The therapist is often asked to participate in more organized games devised by the child and can become a participant in this way in a child's fantasy life. We have already considered in chapter 2 other play activities, such as role playing and concrete exercises, which demand well developed therapeutic skills from the therapist when initiated by children in middle childhood. Other capacities, even a high level of physical stamina, may also prove useful: Tom, age nine, assigned his therapist the role of a famous Argentine soccer player while assigning himself the role of an equally famous English player. Tom simultaneously utilized his intellectual, social and physical skills within this imaginary match. And the therapist found herself challenged in trying to reflect the child's feelings and emotional states while engaged in strenuous physical exercise!

Other more complex symbolic means such as poetry, dance and painting, depending on the child, are also appropriate for representing an older child's experiences. As Wolff states:

Children become poets and painters. They sing and make music. Future writers and artists retain their creativity throughout their lives; most children lose these gifts as adolescence approaches. But for all children their products or athletic skills are a rich source of satisfaction which can compensate for the inevitable failures in other spheres. (1989: 158)

In non-directive play therapy children in middle childhood who have not previously found satisfactions and compensations through symbolic activities can discover these capacities within themselves. And these symbolic expressions can then help sustain them in their often still difficult lives.

ADOLESCENT EMOTIONAL DEVELOPMENT

IDENTITY FORMATION AND NON-DIRECTIVE PLAY THERAPY

In this section we shall discuss non-directive play therapy in relation to early adolescence. During this stage in emotional development childhood play may initially appear to be an inappropriate vehicle for therapeutic engagement; an adult counselling relationship may seem more viable. We shall attempt to demonstrate, however, that non-directive play therapy is an effective and theoretically justifiable means of bridging the stage between childhood and later adolescence/adulthood. In fact, we shall argue that the characteristics of early adolescence itself account for the therapeutic effectiveness of non-directive play therapy at this stage in development.

Historically, adolescence is a relatively new stage in emotional development in our society. For earlier generations, adolescence was nonexistent: childhood ended and adult roles in society were enacted immediately. Now, however, adolescence is a recognizable and acceptable developmental stage, with its own pattern of healthy emotional progression and its own set of problems (Petersen, 1988). Indeed, adolescence is now viewed as a necessary stage of development.

The emotional changes which occur during adolescence are described by Erikson as focusing on identity versus role confusion. 'Identity', as Erikson uses the term, has multiple meanings: first, it describes an adolescent's conscious awareness of individual uniqueness; second, it describes an adolescent's often vague and only half-conscious striving to make sense of past, current and future experience; and third, it describes an adolescent's sense of oneness with society's ideals (Erikson, 1968; Kroger, 1989; Wolff, 1989).

During healthy adolescent development an individual evokes a positive and strong sense of personal uniqueness, along with a commitment to wider society. The negative outcome for this stage, however, is role confusion, an inability to settle on a meaningful personal and societal role. Wolff describes this negative pole as

an indefinitely prolonged uncommitted state in which options are left open, no choices seem inevitable, and the individual fails to acquire a firm sense of who he is, of what he can do, where he is going, with whom, and to what purpose. (1989: 159)

Similarly to other developmental stages, Erikson states that some degree of the negative pole is a necessary part of adolescent emotional development. Without a degree of role confusion, an adolescent may curtail the development of his identity too early, may make his commitment too absolute and not allow himself any flexibility and searching for his adult role in society. As with other developmental progressions, then, although an adolescent does need to develop some degree of role confusion, he needs to develop a preponderance of the positive pole, a sense of his own identity.

For a minority of adolescents, however, role confusion seems to dominate over positive emotional development (Petersen, 1988). Within this period of development, if an adolescent experiences traumatic events or extremely stressful circumstances, a preponderance of negative emotions can develop. John, for example, was universally seen as an extroverted and engaging fourteen-year-old. Following the sudden, and to him completely unforeseen abandonment of the family by his father, to whom John felt emotionally very close, John's personality changed dramatically into that of an introverted, nervous boy with school phobia. When John began attending play therapy sessions, he immediately enacted a short drama using wild animals in which the crocodile fought the bear, won, and dragged the bear off, leaving the other bear alone and unprotected. For several sessions this theme was varied and increasingly personalized and involved the use of different materials, including, finally, puppets. John assigned each puppet a different character with different emotions. They seemed to represent different aspects of his own feelings: the mouse was timid, the bird independent and bossy, the dragon angry and the hedgehog quiet and thoughtful. With these puppets John found a creative play solution to the enactment of abandonment, in which the timid mouse became braver and helped all the animals befriend the dragon. John then seemed able to verbally express to his therapist some of his strong positive and negative feelings about his absent father.

A further reason for John's extreme reaction to his father's abandonment probably was that John was in the process of developing his own sexual identity. With puberty an adolescent develops his adult body size and shape. This brings heightened self-awareness and a realization of his body's new adult permanence, as well as the emergence of new and powerful sexual feelings and emotions. It is necessary for an adolescent to incorporate sexual and emotional changes into the rest of his social and psychological life. He begins to apply adult definitions of a sexual self, influenced by his peers and the media, but also highly influenced by his family and their reactions to his emerging sexual identity (Gagnon, 1972). An adolescent's previous gender role training, as well as his earlier relationships within his family, with his parents in particular, give him guidelines for his new sexual identity. In John's case, his father's sudden abandonment may have called into question for John all his previous and long-held beliefs of appropriate gender role behaviour just at the time that he was tentatively trying out a new adult sexual role himself.

As we will discuss further in the next chapter on sexual abuse, previously developed motor and affective schemas are experimentally applied to new sexual behaviours and new desires for sexual activities by adolescents. Gender role activities which have been learned in childhood – such as control and freedom, the need for achievement and affiliation, aggression and submission – are now applied to the areas of adult sexuality. These gender role schemas must be reapplied and reintegrated and thus develop new meanings. More complex schemas must be developed in relation to the adolescent's own body. For example, childhood schemas of morality related to modesty ("Your mum will chow at you if you don't have any clothes on", as one six-year-old described it), must develop adult meanings; motor schemas which were previously labelled as pure or degrading, good or bad, (say the schemas of kissing or hugging), must be reworked and recreated on an adult level. In addition, an adolescent's schemas related to people must be developed and integrated into earlier schemas on a new adult sexual level. Moral categories such as the distinction between good and bad, and new moral categories, such as the adolescent's moral judgement of, say, homosexuality, may be introduced and need to be developed. In addition, more refined and powerful corresponding motor skills bring the adolescent increased efficacy in his actions and more serious consequences. An adolescent can now enact feelings which previously he had only imagined or wished to enact.

Shifting and powerful emotions, then, can emerge at adolescence which have remained dormant, or even resolved, at an earlier stage in childhood. Problems and emotionally damaging earlier experiences can re-emerge to thwart an adolescent's identity formation, and even precipitate a fresh crisis. Many examples from clinical experience show that as a child develops greater mental and emotional scope in adolescence, he may re-examine painful experiences and feel different and, sometimes, greater distress than he did when the event actually occurred in his childhood. Pynoos and Eth describe, for example, an adolescent they worked with who

witnessed his mother's murder at the age of 7, but has only recently begun to focus on the possible significance of what he views as his mother's flirtatious behaviour. He now concludes that his mother was 'cheating' on her boyfriend and that this was the subject of the fatal argument. (1984: 96)

Other less obviously stressful experiences during childhood can also hinder an adolescent's emotional development. Children who have had numerous discontinuities in their lives, whether caused by parental changes, geographic or economic mobility, or cultural changes (Wolff, 1989), may find it difficult to integrate their past experiences with their current and future life. For example, children who experience discontinuities in parenting may only partially resolve their feelings during their parents' divorce, separation or remarriage and may find that their doubts and confusion assume a more critical and searching quality during adolescence.

Even more difficult is the task for adopted or fostered children who may feel largely cut off from their past and unable to integrate their early experiences into their identity at adolescence, partly because of lack of information (or mis-information) about themselves during childhood. Without adults to serve as a repository of memories during childhood, they may feel inadequate to or frustrated by having to rely completely on their own partial and incomplete memories. Another facet of identity these adolescents may be missing is a knowledge of their own parents. Part of the resolution of the question of "Who am I?" lies in examining who one's parents are. By taking a wider view of their parents, adolescents can reject, accept or sift through parental attributes and gain a wider perspective and, even, mental strategies for developing into the people they are and want to become.

Sarah, age sixteen, was emotionally abused and rejected by her mother when she was six years old. She was later adopted by a middle-aged couple who led a highly circumscribed social life. During play therapy sessions Sarah did not directly examine her past rejection by her mother or the introversion of her adoptive parents. Instead she slowly and hesitantly, while painting and drawing, began to explore her painful sense of missing out on friendships with both boys and girls due to her paralysing shyness and fear of rejection. Towards the end of her play therapy sessions Sarah was accepted for entry at a sixth form college for the following year. She became determined to change into the kind of person she wished to become, and discussed her resolve to master her shyness with the therapist. Sarah also wistfully acknowledged that she was uncertain how to do this and wished someone could help her practise, so she wouldn't fail. The therapist reflected her feelings of uncertainty, hopefulness and determination; she then suggested to Sarah that perhaps Sarah would like to work with the therapist in her last sessions jointly to develop and role play social strategies for handling situations she anticipated she would find most difficult.

Sarah's creative solution to her shyness illustrates how not just on a physical and emotional level, but on an intellectual level as well, adolescence is a period of rapid growth and change. At this stage in cognitive development an adolescent's thought processes change qualitatively. Rather than needing concrete objects and experiences to reach accurate solutions to problems as he did earlier, an adolescent now begins to work out abstract solutions mentally, without recourse to direct experience (Piaget, 1967). Most adolescents, as Sarah did, can think more abstractly about imagined or logically possible events, can explore possible alternative solutions to problems systematically and think more objectively about their own thought processes than younger children. They are also more able to extend their personal horizon to include not only past events but future possibilities. Adolescents, when compared with younger children, are more likely to develop strategies and individual rules for processing information and solving both practical and theoretical problems. In addition, they have increased memory capacity and an increased attention to detail that most younger children lack (Flavell, 1985). These cognitive changes, then, enable an adolescent to have a wider range of intellectual capacities. An adolescent, because of his increased mental and physical maturity, needs to counterpoint his own personality against his parents and against his childhood self. Discontinuities of development, as we have illustrated, make this task more difficult. Non-directive play therapy can be an effective therapeutic means for integrating past experiences into healthy identity development. The adolescent who comes to therapy may have developed a preponderance of the negative pole in any of the earlier stages in his emotional development. Because the adolescent can choose to direct the sessions to suit his own current needs, his negative earlier experiences may emerge in a variety of ways.

An adolescent who has developed a preponderance of mistrust of parents, school, police, etc. may be unable to commit himself to any people or institutions. He may feel a strong cynical mistrust, along with a feeling of everything being arbitrary and unpredictable. Nothing may seem worthwhile enough to commit himself to, to risk an identification with. Or an adolescent may feel himself to be too trusting of adults and unable to make reasoned judgements; in defence he may vehemently reject all adults and all adult institutions. Because he realizes that he cannot choose the good and reject the bad aspects of people and institutions in a working relationship, he may decide to make an all-or-none commitment.

These basic emotional conflicts centring around trust may emerge immediately in the therapist's sessions with an adolescent and therapy may focus primarily on the adolescent's mistrust of the therapist and his mistrust of the therapeutic process. As with younger children, the therapist would reflect and empathize with the adolescent's feelings of mistrust of herself and her work; and most of the sessions may be devoted to this theme.

The second stage of emotional development, autonomy versus shame and doubt, may also emerge in therapeutic work with adolescents. Non-directive play therapy, as we shall discuss more fully in the last part of the chapter, is pre-eminently suited to this kind of conflict. An adolescent not only strongly desires autonomy in his personal life, say in choosing his own clothes, friends and academic programme, but also wants to have the autonomy to develop his own set of values. If he feels his autonomy has been aborted in the past, from over restraint by parents or school, or a lack of constraint and a laissez-faire attitude by carers, or by being criticized and blamed unduly when he made common mistakes, the adolescent may have difficulty feeling autonomy and free will in adolescence. He may feel strongly that it is preferable to have a negative identity because he was able to choose it himself, rather than an identity forced on him by his parents, his school or society. Acting a part, feeling he is 'not real' can, for an adolescent, be a source of deep shame and doubt in himself. Unfortunately, an adolescent may find that his perhaps temporary hostile identity has real and negative consequences for acceptance in adult society (Wolff, 1989). By being defined negatively, say in police records, the adolescent may find that he cannot easily escape the label imposed on him (even in his adulthood) and it may have negative implications in, for example, limiting his choice of a career.

Other labels, more directly related to therapeutic work, may also adversely affect identity formation during adolescence. Some adolescents would strongly resent therapeutic help if they believed they were risking being labelled 'nutty' by their families, peers or adult society. Indeed, sometimes effective therapeutic intervention must be balanced by the danger of stigmatizing an adolescent further who already shows role confusion. An example is Patricia, age thirteen, who was very reluctant to attend play therapy sessions required by the court and extremely distrustful of the therapist initially. The beginning sessions centred on her feelings of anger, resentment and fear over being coerced into a relationship with the therapist that she perceived only in negative terms. Her greatest fear, as she confided later on in her play therapy sessions, had been that she would be called "bonkers", as her aunt had been, all the rest of her life.

With the third stage of emotional development, initiative versus guilt, an adolescent takes the attitudes he has developed in childhood towards future adult roles and towards self-initiated activities and applies these attitudes in exploring his position in adult society. In comparison with most adults, an adolescent will normally have wide ambitions for himself in adult society and feel a need to explore different possible work roles. He will also want to take the initiative in forming different kinds of personal relationships with fellow adolescents and with adult men and women. Above all, he does not want his ambitions stifled until he has the opportunity to explore some of them himself.

Jerry, age fourteen, was referred for play therapy because of his stealing, housebreaking and violence towards other adolescents. When Jerry began exploring his frustrations with his current life, he began to express anger over how "unfair" everything was in his life. He displayed high intelligence and advanced motor skills, as well as numerous ambitions. Yet he repeatedly referred to different ideas he had tried to implement – building a go-cart, designing an adventure playground "for kids of all sizes", making a dirt track in a disused field "for everyone to use" – which had been stifled and had to be abandoned because of a lack of adult encouragement and commitment. His creative contributions towards society were never realized or appreciated. As therapy progressed Jerry explored with the therapist other acceptable ways to gain recognition for his positive feelings and develop his skills.

If, unlike Jerry, an adolescent has developed a preponderance of guilt from past emotional development, he may react by role fixation and a constriction of his ambitions because he is afraid to venture into the adult world (Wolff, 1989). Or he may react by denying all guilt and attempt to lead a guilt-free delinquency. In the next chapter on sexual abuse, examples will be given of abused adolescents who either constricted their lives in order to ensure their safety or attempted to deny all guilt feelings by their delinquency.

The last stage in emotional development prior to adolescence, industry versus inferiority, and the ensuing sense of competence that emerges with a preponderance of industry, must also be reintegrated by the adolescent into the adult work role. If school and family experiences have enhanced a child's sense of self-esteem, he can imagine himself more easily in a competent adult work role. However, if self-esteem is undermined by school and family experiences, both work paralysis and social withdrawal can occur. Erikson states that the "inability to settle on an occupational identity is what most disturbs young people" (1968: 132) An adolescent wants a meaningful job, both meaningful to himself and one which society itself defines as "meaningful". This concern is often acknowledged by an adolescent in therapy sessions and he is sometimes able to examine with the therapist different future career possibilities.

We shall now consider in more detail specific practice issues in working therapeutically with this age group. One of the main obstacles that both the therapist and the adolescent himself must overcome in employing non-directive play therapy during early adolescence is that, on the face of it, the adolescent might seem much too old for most of the play materials in the room. It is important for the therapist to be aware of the uneasiness that might exist in many adolescents (and, at times in somewhat younger children) when confronted with "a roomful of baby toys". Care must be taken by the therapist to structure the encounter so that the adolescent feels a sense of permissive-ness, as would a younger child, while ensuring, in addition, that the adolescent senses that his age is being respected. Because he is unsure of his status himself, which is, as we discussed, somewhere between childhood and adulthood, he can be unusually sensitive to situations which attempt to treat him only as a child. But since he is not an adult, an office used for counselling adults without any play materials present will seem unsuitable in most cases and it can be both intimidating and 'boring'.

More specifically, the therapist in non-directive play therapy can overcome an adolescent's initial unease by structuring both the materials in the room with older children in mind and by structuring her introduction to the room to suit an adolescent. Some materials seem particularly suited to older childhood and early adolescence: clay can be intricately modelled and painted or manipulated while talking; soft balls can be kicked around or used in organized games; playing cards can be used for magic tricks, building a house of cards or card games with the therapist; puppets can have stages made and scripts written for them; paints, pens, pencils, and other drawing materials can be used for symbolic representations; sets of small farm animals, people, cars, bricks and trees can be used to create intricate symbolic layouts of reality.

Other materials may suggest themselves to the adolescent as play therapy progresses. For example, one adolescent was modelling with playdough and repeatedly regretted that there weren't several colours of playdough, rather than just one to use, and became frustrated by the limited use of the material she had. After reflecting the adolescent's feelings a few times, the therapist brought in three more colours for the next session. The adolescent creatively mixed playdoughs together to make still more colours and was then able to model realistic-looking fruits, cakes, pastries and breads, which the adolescent found aesthetically very pleasing, a positive emotion which was reflected back to the adolescent by the therapist.

In addition to selecting some materials appropriate for older children and adolescents, the therapist can also structure the play therapy room itself to include older ages of children. By having easy chairs as well as play materials, the therapist will be able to demonstrate to the adolescent on entering the play therapy room that it is used by children of all different ages to both sit and talk in and play in, and that he is free to make use of whatever is in the room. By structuring the play sessions permissively and sensitively, the therapist will be able to engage most adolescents, in spite of their reluctance to look 'babyish' to outsiders. Ensuring confidentiality and privacy also helps break down adolescents' reservations about being with children's toys.

Once the adolescent trusts the situation and the therapist to some degree, the advantages of using non-directive play therapy will become apparent. First, as stated earlier with younger children, play materials can be used to give symbolic expression to an adolescent's past and current problems. As symbols, they can be a less threatening means to express personal problems, as well as being meaningful ways in themselves to convey multi-dimensional experiences. Because an adolescent has more complex and abstract mental abilities than younger children, he may consciously understand his symbolic expressions more fully than a younger child would and use them consciously to make sense of his inner world. With non-directive play therapy the therapist attempts to reflect these expressed feelings and thoughts back to the adolescent, using the symbolic means he chooses himself for working on his perceived (or half-perceived) problems.

The second major advantage in using non-directive play therapy with adolescents is that the situation itself easily permits the adolescent to work on reintegrating his experiences into his current life and thoughts. More so than for children, an adolescent is cut off and prohibited from using children's toys and behaviour. By using materials suitable for differing ages of children, the adolescent will be more easily reminded of different stages in his own development. Especially for adolescents who have experienced childhood discontinuities, traumas or stresses as illustrated earlier, integrating difficult past experiences into their identity is an essential component of therapeutic work. Adolescents in non-directive play therapy, then, can suck the baby's bottle, use finger paints, role play and so on, much as younger children do when they relive their past experiences. And unlike other more directive methods, the adolescent can choose his own appropriate materials and the appropriate time for their use, without outside pressure.

This self-direction is essential during adolescence. As we stated above, an adolescent strives for autonomy in his personal and communal life. If he feels unduly pressured from outside, he may feel unable to live his 'real self'. In non-directive play therapy, while the therapist still sets appropriate limits, necessarily broader than given to younger children, the majority of decisions during the session are left to the adolescent. Problems in an adolescent's current functioning which relate to autonomy are thus immediately experienced and addressed within the therapeutic relationship, as are the other areas of adolescent difficulties mentioned above of trust, initiative and industry.

The other important dimension to consider in non-directive play therapy with adolescents is that the adolescent is in the process of forming his identity in relation to the adult world. The therapist in the therapeutic relationship represents the adult world in a very direct sense for the adolescent. More than with younger children, the adolescent challenges and tries to understand the worker's personality, values and place in society. If the therapist herself has a sense of role confusion and an unstable value hierarchy, she will necessarily fail to help the adolescent find his own identity and value system. As we discussed above, it is by counterpointing his own personality and values to others that the adolescent finds his own identity.

Janet, age fifteen, had grown up in a highly sexualized family atmosphere in which adult–child role boundaries in many areas, including sexual relations, were blurred; this atmosphere had existed in the family for several generations. When Janet began to attend play therapy, she had extremely mixed feelings towards her family, from whom she had been separated because of the continuing risk of sexual abuse. Because her family often distorted and failed to discuss important events in her life, the key issue in the initial sessions for Janet was whether the therapist would be a reliable and trustworthy person. Janet tested the worker's trustworthiness in several ways: by testing the confidentiality of her own sessions; by testing it in relation to other children in play therapy; and by testing it in relation to other professionals. Janet often asked about other children and what they did, what their problems were, and expressed a genuine desire to meet them and share experiences with them. The therapist stressed her need strictly to maintain her rule of confidentiality for Janet's sessions. The therapist also reiterated that she had to maintain silence on other children in spite of Janet's genuine and understandable interest in them. The therapist reflected Janet's feelings back to her as well as clearly stating her own position in each instance and giving reasons for her stand to Janet. With this approach by the therapist, Janet seemed to become able to focus more directly on her own values and how they differed from both her family's and the worker's values.

Janet's use of her initial sessions illustrates another aspect of work with adolescents that can differ from non-directive play therapy with younger children. Because an adolescent is in the process of becoming an adult, the therapist often finds that she vacillates between an adult non-directive counselling role and a play therapy role. But as in work with younger children, the adolescent himself determines whether a verbal or nonverbal means (or a combination) is the most suitable method to work on his problems. The therapist must be prepared with adolescents, however, to have developed sufficient counselling skills on an adult level to be effective in working with adolescents when they choose this approach. Talking through problems is a chosen method not just for adolescents, but for younger children as well, to some extent. However with adolescence, as we discussed above, the ability verbally and symbolically to express complex thought will often have taken on the majority of adult characteristics.

6

Sexual Abuse and Non-directive Play Therapy

Many of the feelings and difficulties the sexually abused child experiences are similar in nature to those faced by all children referred for therapeutic help: coming to terms with being 'referred' at all, for children and adolescents rarely request therapeutic help even when they are aware of its availability; being viewed by others as either having or being 'a problem'; the discomfort of explaining painful, embarrassing, sensitive feelings that have rarely, if ever, been revealed, or indeed consciously acknowledged by the child himself; knowing that an adult and initially a stranger as well, is writing down or recording the very things which expose the child, or make him feel vulnerable; risking himself with another, to be prepared to expend time and energy, thought and imagination in explaining his world in the presence of his therapist. These are all aspects of therapy which each child at some stage will need to address. They make understandable the apprehension with which children approach therapeutic sessions, and are of particular relevance when working therapeutically with a sexually abused child.

Sexual abuse has been described in its effect as most akin to severe emotional abuse. Glaser and Frosh state that "in general, and except in instances of associated physical injury or rape by strangers, child sexual abuse is best classed alongside severe emotional abuse in terms of its structure and effects". (1988: 9) It does, however, have certain characteristics which make it clearly distinct from emotional or physical abuse, although it may contain elements of both.

One such distinction is the abuser's intentional distortion of the child's reality. Because the abuser tries constantly to present the sexually abusive relationship as 'normal', enormous conflicts and confusions are created for the child who must endeavour to integrate his inner experience of the abuse with the abuser's presentation of reality. The abuser may describe the relationship in terms of 'special and loving' and the experience of sexual abuse as something the child should find pleasurable and good, which is at times different from the child's inner experience.

Another dimension is that the relationship must be kept secret at all costs. This additional, heightened emphasis on secrecy, whilst also present in some physically abusive episodes, is an essential component of sexual abuse if it is to continue. It is crucial that the abuser achieves and maintains the silence of the child throughout the abusive experience, which may continue for many years. An additional element, now closely associated with sexual abuse, is its compulsive nature (Furniss, 1991; Wyre and Smith, 1990). Work in the recent past, such as that of Wyre and Smith (1990) and Giaretto (1982) with sexual offenders, has informed therapeutic intervention and confronted the long-held myth of the 'one-off' offender or the incestuous offender, as opposed to the paedophile. The sexually abused child may mirror the compulsive nature of the sexual abuse in his own sexualized behaviour. The repeated sexual arousal of the child and the resulting tension created by the abuse may lead the child to find relief through his own sexual stimulation, either alone or with the involvement of others.

Another distinctive characteristic of sexual abuse is that it distorts the child's relationship with the abuser, particularly when the latter is the primary attachment figure for the child and has the role of provider of his emotional and physical care. It also distorts the child's view of other significant relationships and his view of himself; the sexual abuse interrupts and damages the child's subsequent emotional development from the onset of the abuse.

We shall look in some detail at the impact sexual abuse is likely to have on the child's emotional development in the next part of the chapter. We shall then turn to a brief consideration of the symptomology of the sexually abused child. Since sexual abuse may not have been diagnosed before the therapeutic work began (an issue we discuss more fully in the next chapter), it is important for the therapist to have a good understanding of the symptomology of the sexually abused child. However, since the focus of this book is on therapeutic intervention, rather than on either the assessment of possible abuse or on the complex aetiology of individual cases, our discussion of symptomology here is necessarily brief and the reader is referred elsewhere for a more detailed consideration of the subject. The third part of the chapter will explore some of the particular issues and themes which may emerge during non-directive play therapy or counselling with the sexually abused child. These issues will include characteristic feelings of the child, his sexualized behaviour, self-mutilation and dissociative reactions. Finally we shall discuss those issues in working with sexually abused children which are more directly relevant to the therapist herself.

As a preliminary to our discussion of emotional development we should state at the outset that we consider child sexual abuse to be emotionally damaging. The majority of children and adults who have been victims of child sexual abuse report negative feelings related to their abuse. The emotional damage to the child may be serious and have long-term consequences if therapeutic help, in addition to the support and belief of those closest to the child, is not available. Finkelhor concludes that

from clinical and non-clinical populations the findings concerning the trauma of child sexual abuse appear to be as follows – in the immediate aftermath of sexual abuse one-fifth to two-fifths of abused children seen by clinicians manifest some noticeable disturbance ... when studied as adults. Victims as a group demonstrate more impairment than their non-victimized counterparts (about twice as much) but less than one-fifth evidence serious psychopathology. These findings give reassurance to victims that extreme long-term effects are not inevitable ... [however] ... they also suggest that risk of initial and long-term mental health impairment for victims of child sexual abuse should be taken very seriously. (Finkelhor et al., 1986: 164)

The difficulty in clinical work lies in determining what particular damage the sexual abuse is likely to have for each individual child in a unique sense and then in determining whether this emotional damage can be mitigated by therapeutic intervention.

THE RELATIONSHIP OF SEXUAL ABUSE TO EMOTIONAL DEVELOPMENT

In reviewing the impact child sexual abuse has on the child's emotional development, we shall use Erikson's stages of emotional development delineated in the previous chapter to form a conceptual framework for the discussion.

It has been noted earlier that each stage brings with it the potential for both positive and negative development. Sexual abuse, because of its negative and distorting effect on the child's emotional growth may, as Finkelhor suggests, seriously damage or interrupt this process and result in long-term mental health difficulties, if not addressed therapeutically.

The child's development of trust versus mistrust during infancy may be interrupted or blocked if sexual abuse begins at this time. Even when the abuse has not been by the child's primary carer, but rather within the context of the child's family, the child's development of trust with his mother or father may nevertheless be damaged. For the greater part of childhood he is emotionally and physically dependent on his carers, and on their ability to protect him from harm. In particular the child requires consistency of parental care. The presence of an attachment figure and the quality of care offered enables the child to achieve, on balance, a feeling of basic trust. Where this has never been achieved, or has been interrupted, it will have damaging later consequences for the child. Two examples will illustrate this point.

Jeffrey, age two and a half, had been removed from home one year earlier because of his parents' abuse of him and his older sister. Jeffrey was referred for therapy when he failed to develop a close relationship with his foster parents over the year, especially with his foster father, despite their kindness and concern for him. This mistrust permeated every area of his life: he could not tolerate being held by either foster parent, with his body becoming rigid when he was in close proximity to them; he always refused help with his food, struggling to feed himself at times rather than letting himself be helped; and he became most anxious and agitated, his foster parents related, when he was lying down, especially when his nappy was being changed.

The therapist had twelve sessions with Jeffrey and included the anatomically correct family of dolls (with their clothes remaining on) in her play equipment as she was concerned about the possibility of Jeffrey having been sexually abused. Because of his age and his great mistrust, the therapist worked at Jeffrey's foster home, with the full co-operation of the foster parents. The most significant session for Jeffrey, and a turning point in his therapy and in his relationship to his foster parents, occurred in the ninth session.

This session, similarly to the others, was largely non-verbal. Jeffrey indicated that the therapist was to hold the largest male doll (the 'father' figure), as usual, but then he suddenly became angry with the doll and snatched it from the therapist, banging the doll's head repeatedly on the floor and shouting. He then asked for nappy cream and put the cream repeatedly on the therapist's cheeks and face, especially around the mouth area. The therapist felt that the manner in which Jeffrey rubbed cream into her face and put his finger around her lips had sexual connotations, and responded, as he pushed his finger in and out of her mouth, that it was nice for Jeffrey but not nice for her.

Then Jeffrey insisted that the therapist change his nappy and put cream on him. She changed his nappy and he became physically relaxed and smiling, then lay down on the sofa and sucked a baby bottle filled with orange juice, looking serene and peaceful.

That night, Jeffrey awoke his foster father after midnight and told him in detail about the sexual abuse he had experienced with both his natural parents. Later, having returned to sleep, he then woke up his foster mother and repeated to her the same account of his abusive experiences. From the next morning onwards, Jeffrey was able to initiate affectionate behaviour towards both his foster parents. He began spontaneously to hold their hands, to ask to go with one or other of them in the car, and remained calm while his nappy was changed.

Jeffrey seemed to have had a distorted and abusive relationship with his parents perhaps from his earliest months of life. As Helen demonstrated in our earlier chapter, Jeffrey appeared in some way to know what a healthy relationship with adults should consist of and was able immediately and matter-of-factly to live out an emotionally normal life after he had re-enacted his abusive experience during play therapy. The permanent affective schemas he had developed in a distorted way with his natural parent seemed to be radically transformed and shifted once re-enactment of abuse had occurred. It also, incidentally, made him free to verbalize his preverbal abusive experiences at his current level of mental functioning and language development.

Finally, it seems clear from this example that a highly compensatory environment may not be enough for a child in order to transform his permanent affective schemas. Although this compensatory environment is a necessary precondition, the child also seems to need to re-enact his emotionally damaging experience on a symbolic level. Perhaps this is because the shift must be actively initiated by the child and it must involve affective, cognitive and motor schemas in an internal, radical transformation.

Another example of this type of distortion in emotional development was manifest in therapeutic work with Jane, age fifteen years. This first stage of trust versus mistrust had never been satisfactorily achieved during her early emotional development. Jane had been a much wanted baby, however her premature and difficult delivery, coupled with her mother's disappointment at having a girl, resulted in her mother's early rejection and subsequent abandonment of her. Her father became her prime carer and sexually abused Jane through her middle childhood and into adolescence. Central to Jane's feelings of mistrust of others and of herself was her fundamentally damaged relationship with her mother, whom she felt had betrayed her when she was most helpless and vulnerable. She felt that if her mother could have let her down so profoundly, there was little hope of finding anyone else she could trust in. The early damage resulting from her mother's rejection of her was compounded by her father's subsequent sexual abuse.

Even where the establishment of basic trust has been laid as a foundation, it may not be a lasting achievement. Trust can be impaired during later development if the child experiences sexual abuse. The child is likely to feel a sense of deprivation and abandonment by his carer(s) even when they have not been directly involved in the abuse.

The sexually abused child may also have a sense of mistrust of himself, of his feelings and of his own body. This mistrust may be particularly apparent when the child has felt some physical pleasure during the sexual abuse, or where he has a strong emotional attachment and loyalty to his abuser. Even where the sexual abuse has been extremely damaging, it may nonetheless have been within the context of the child's most significant relationship.

The therapeutic relationship will mirror to a significant degree the child's functioning in other relationships. He may have insufficient trust in the therapist and be unable to engage successfully in the process of therapy itself: this inability to engage in therapy is especially pertinent to adolescence, which we shall discuss shortly. In general, however, the therapeutic and enabling attitudes of empathy, acceptance and congruence will usually lead to a decrease in the child's defensiveness, thus enabling him to begin to establish a feeling of trust with the therapist. This is a basic requirement if the therapeutic relationship is to be an enabling one.

The experience of the therapist as a consistent, warm, trustworthy adult, offers the child a new opportunity to explore more appropriate ways of relating to others. The child's deep mistrust can be mitigated by a relationship with an adult who does not invade or abuse him as the perpetrator has done, or inadequately protect or blame him as the non-abusing parent may have done. Once trust has been established, the child will discover that the adult (therapist) does not

---

sexualize this intimate and caring relationship, contrary to his previous relationship with the abuser and contrary perhaps also to his negative relationship with his other, non-abusing parent. The therapeutic relationship, in valuing the child for himself, without any expectations or wish for a sexual response, will provide the child with a contrasting experience against which to compare the abusive relationship. The sexual abuse may have deprived the child of his basic emotional needs over a long period of time. Consequently, he may enter the therapeutic relationship desperate for attention and/or affection and overly willing to place his trust in the therapist from the outset. By doing this, in other circumstances, the child may well become vulnerable to further exploitation since he will not have developed enough mistrust to protect himself against further abuse.

Sexual abuse experienced during the next developmental stage of autonomy versus shame and doubt may also result in unhealthy emotional development. It may either induce a disproportionate sense of shame and doubt in the child, or threaten an older child's already established sense of autonomy. The child's wish for choice vies with his need for protection from meaningless and arbitrary experiences of doubt during this period. The sexually abused child has usually been given many false messages about his own autonomy. The child, in fact, has no real choice at any stage about rejecting the abuse, and has no control over the feelings of shame and doubt that may result. Such feelings are frequently encouraged in the child by the perpetrator, for along with them the child also feels a sense of responsibility for having allowed the abuse to take place, or a responsibility at least at having participated in the abuse. This sense of responsibility and a feeling of having been an active participant is frequently used to silence the child.

Partly because of this, those working with sexually abused children need to be cautious when addressing the issue of the child protecting himself in the future. A child is unlikely to be able to say 'no' to sexual abuse in many situations and, indeed, in doing so may put himself at greater risk. The abused child may also have been encouraged to view his behaviour as seductive by the perpetrator who is then able to disown responsibility for the abuse which follows. Implying to the child that he has the ability to say no may exacerbate his sense of responsibility. He can, however, be helped to identify situations and behaviour which might become abusive and to identify a safe, reliable and readily available adult to turn to if he is troubled.

Alternatively, the sexual abuse may have been used as a punishment for, say, his behaviour at wetting or soiling. The child's feelings of shame and self-consciousness can be greatly heightened by his sexual abuse. Erikson comments "there is a limit to a child's ... endurance in the face of demands to consider himself, his body and his wishes as evil and dirty". (1977: 227) Damage at this stage of development may be the forerunner of compulsive self-doubt which can become particularly acute during adolescence, if not resolved by earlier therapeutic help. In healthy emotional development the child develops a sense of self-control without the loss of self-esteem; from this stems a lasting sense of his own goodwill and pride. When the child is sexually abused he both feels the loss of self-control and experiences excessive control from others. This brings with it a lasting feeling of shame and doubt. These feelings are often noted as amongst the most intensely negative feelings described by victims of child sexual abuse (Haugaard and Reppucci, 1988).

The therapeutic implications of the child's feelings of loss of self-control must be considered carefully at the referral stage. Often the child has no choice about whether he attends therapy or not. This is particularly the case when a therapeutic intervention has been ordered by the court. If this lack of choice is not honestly explored by the therapist at the outset it is likely to reinforce the earlier damage to the child and increase his confusion.

Whilst the child may have no choice about his attendance at play therapy sessions, within this therapeutic approach he does have real choices regarding activities and conversations. The re-establishment of choice and autonomy then, particularly for victims of child sexual abuse, is extremely important and can be therapeutically addressed in an immediate and direct way in non-directive play therapy.

In describing the therapeutic contact with women who were sexually abused as children, Jehu explores the issue of control and choice:

There is a tendency to actively resist being influenced by others. When a client perceives herself as having some choice, and that this choice is being restricted, threatened or eliminated by the therapist, then the client will tend to experience discomfort and strive to restore the lost freedom. Because of their history of domination and exploitation by others, victims of sexual abuse may be especially on guard against external influence. (Jehu et al., 1989: 40)

During the third stage of initiative versus guilt the child develops a sense of purpose and direction in his actions. The preliminary negative emotion developed during this period is the child's sense of guilt over the goals he has contemplated or initiated. If sexual abuse begins at this stage of his development, the child may experience overwhelming guilt, particularly as he is likely to feel responsible for some, if not all, of the sexual abuse that has occurred. Like shame and doubt, guilt may also be exacerbated by the professional response to the child's sexual abuse, particularly at the investigatory stage. Interviewers may ask why the child waited passively for the perpetrator to return and re-abuse him? Why the child went into the perpetrator's bedroom knowing that he would be abused? Why did he not tell anyone or try to stop the abuse in some other way? Yet the child would not have been able to control either the perpetrator's or his own actions to this degree.

If the abuse began before this stage, guilt is unlikely to be such a major issue for the child. The young child would know and accept that he was in a dependent relationship with the abuser and had to obey. Whilst a younger child might feel confusion over his sexual abuse, he is less likely to feel responsible for it in the same way that an older child might. We wish to clarify here that while in general we reject Freudian psychosexual mechanisms in explaining normal emotional development, the sexual elements of Freudian theory may be more true in some ways for the sexually abused child than in children experiencing healthy emotional development. One example, among many, from Erikson states that the child during the initiative versus guilt stage experiences "intensified fear of finding . . . the genitals harmed as a punishment for the fantasies attached to their excitement". (1977: 230) This may indeed be the experience of the child who suffers the physical damage to himself consequent upon penetrative assault.

The fourth stage of development, industry versus inferiority, may also be distorted by the experience of sexual abuse. The negative side of this stage for the child is the development of a preponderance of inadequacy and inferiority. The sexual abuse may make the child feel inferior in several ways. An older child's peer group becomes increasingly important, but a sexually abused child is likely to feel isolated and different from his contemporaries because his own sexual experiences are so far removed from those of his friends. Sue, for example, found it hard to share the excitement of her friends when they were discussing the experience of a first kiss, having been subjected to sexual intercourse by her father for a number of years.

The perpetrator may also endeavour to increase the child's isolation, keeping him away from peer group friendships, because of jealousy or because the perpetrator is fearful that the child might disclose the sexual abuse if he develops intimate peer friendships (Salter, 1988). Jill, for instance, was not allowed to use the telephone, to invite her friends home, or to have boyfriends until her late adolescence. Even then, her stepfather would fly into a rage if a boy telephoned her at home. (This response may be particularly characteristic of male abusers.)

If the child's normal emotional development is interrupted at this stage by sexual abuse, it may result in the child under-achieving, either because he is unable to establish the emotional space required for intellectual growth or because the concerns of older childhood seem so far removed from his own life experiences. The child may begin to mirror the perpetrator by having the whole focus of his existence revolve around the next abusive episode; he may also experience feelings of stress, anxiety, fear, dread and avoidance. He may despair of his ability or may not be free to invest in it because of lack of concentration or preoccupation with the abuse. Feelings of isolation and separation from his peer group may easily develop because of his very different experiences. He may then either lose or fail to develop his sense of identity in relation to them.

Conversely the child may try to overachieve at school, in an attempt to regain some control over his life, which he lacks so greatly by being abused. It may provide a way for the child to become or feel he is superior and therefore compensate for some of the damage to his peer group relationships created by the sexual abuse. The recognition of his intellectual abilities therefore becomes a compensation for the other traumas in the child's life. School may in these circumstances provide a safe and encouraging haven for the child (unless, as in some unfortunate cases, the abuse is actually taking place there). The child in achieving academically experiences success and hope which counteracts the feelings of despair, hopelessness and helplessness engendered by the abuse. However, if the child makes a heavy investment in success at school and fails, the damage will then be intensified.

The fifth stage of identity versus role confusion is also adversely affected by sexual abuse. In adolescence, as we discussed in the previous chapter, all the sameness and continuities relied on in earlier childhood are questioned and re-evaluated. The adolescent is concerned about how he appears to others in contrast to what he feels he is. Sexual abuse, bringing with it feelings of low self-esteem, anger, confusion, isolation, self-disgust and stigmatization, interrupts and damages this exploration. If the abuse is continuing, the adolescent's attempts to rework the issues of earlier years will be thwarted. Erikson notes that "the danger of this stage is role confusion where this is based on a strong previous doubt as to one's sexual identity". (1977: 235) This of course has far reaching implications for the sexually abused child; where the child rejects the role of the perpetrator (male) and also the role of the non-protecting parent (female) there may be no one left for him to identify with. As Erikson and other psychoanalytic writers suggest, the child needs to be able to love his parents and to have some identification with them in order to further his emotional development.

Andrea, for example, had been sexually abused from an early age by her mother's three successive cohabitees. During those times when her mother had not been in a relationship, she had turned to Andrea to take over the role of partnering her. Andrea had been expected to look after her mother, whose health was poor, from a very young age. She was also given the responsibility of disciplining her young brother and sister. Whilst she had enjoyed the status and special place in the family which this role had conferred on her, she had also found it confusing. She was particularly bitter and resentful when the third cohabitee joined the family. Equally confusing were her new feelings of affection for this man when he began to sexually abuse her. Shortly after her placement outside the family, she became involved in a lesbian relationship which resulted in her mother's further rejection of her.

The adolescent looking towards the future can view academic success, where they have attained it, as a way out of the abusing family. As they view the future, particularly adult identity and the role they may have in that future, many sexually abused young people identify with certain professions, in particular social work and the police. This identification may be a healthy adjustment to their own abuse, and sometimes a realistic career choice later (provided that they have already worked through personal issues for themselves), since they see in these occupations the opportunity to protect children as they wish they had been protected in their own childhoods. In being able to envisage being in an occupation which embues the individual with success, power and control, they can see themselves regaining the power and control in their own lives. This pattern was demonstrated by Olive, age sixteen and Maggie, age thirteen. They had been removed from their family some years before therapeutic work began because their stepfather had sexually abused Olive. The abuse of Maggie had only just begun when Olive disclosed that she was being abused. Olive had decided on a career as a social worker; Maggie hoped to become a police cadet.

Sexual experimentation is a normal part of development for adolescents. If, as a result of sexual abuse normal sexual inhibitions and boundaries are not in place, the young person may turn to the sexual abuse of other children. This albeit damaging behaviour for both the abused child and the abusive adolescent perhaps has the function of allowing the adolescent to re-enact the trauma of the abuse and, in so doing, try to regain some control over it. It also gives him the opportunity to evaluate other children's reaction to the abuse and compare it to his own. It is further damaging for the abusing adolescent when he is apprehended and the long-term consequences of such experimentation preclude a healthier future. (We shall return to this issue in the fourth part of the chapter.) Role playing in non-directive play therapy serves this function of re-enactment without these damaging consequences.

Adolescence also involves the experience of 'falling in love' which is partly an attempt to arrive at a definition of identity by projecting a diffused sense of self on to another. By seeing its reflection a gradual clarification of self may emerge. Where peer group contact is jealously ruled out by the perpetrator, this opportunity as well is blocked.

The adolescent in therapy can begin to explore healthy and meaningful ways to come to terms with the sexual abuse and its consequences. He can begin the process of integration of what has happened to him with his view of the future, and his adult functioning in that future. Within the therapeutic relationship his coping mechanisms can be explored and lead to healthy growth rather than dysfunction. The adolescent is also given a different role model of a caring, consistent, non-judgemental adult. At times the contrast between the therapist and the person who abused the adolescent, who may often have been the parent, is too painfully stark for the young person to tolerate, and he may withdraw from therapy.

In conclusion, we have considered the implications sexual abuse is likely to have for the emotional development of the child at some length because, as stated earlier, the possibility of damage to, or distortion of, the child's develop-ment appears to be a real consequence of sexual abuse. The abuse can create distortion at any stage in the child's development; in addition, earlier stages which have been successfully negotiated may well be disrupted.

For adolescents there exists the additional possibility of emotional distress as they look back to their childhood and feel an increased sense of guilt, believing they could have stopped the abuse or disclosed it at an earlier stage. In reality, because of their dependent relationship on the abuser, this would not have been a viable option for the child, even though from their current vantage point in adolescence they may now imagine that they had more options than existed in fact.

THE SYMPTOMOLOGY OF SEXUAL ABUSE

The therapist, in addition to having an understanding of how sexual abuse affects emotional development, also needs an awareness of symptoms the sexually abused child may exhibit in therapy. The child may not have been recognized as sexually abused prior to referral and the possibility of disclosure of abuse during therapy needs to be kept in mind. The therapist is also more likely to provide accurate reflection, empathy and a congruent use of her own feelings if she has a sound knowledge of the likely effect of sexual abuse on the child.

The recognition of sexual abuse has focused largely on the emotional and behavioural sequelae that have come to be associated with the sexually abused child. This has been a notably different approach from physical abuse, where little attention has been given to the emotional consequences of the abuse, and far greater emphasis placed on the nature of the child's injuries. As a consequence physical abuse has remained largely in the domain of the consultant physician or paediatrician. In contrast, sexual abuse has remained in the province of psychiatrists and, until the Cleveland Inquiry (Butler-Sloss, 1988) the involvement of paediatricians was less noticeable. The reason behind this rather different response from the medical profession is an obvious one – whilst the diagnosis of physical abuse relies heavily on the medical evidence, the diagnosis of sexual abuse is different. Glaser and Frosh argue that

Fewer than half the children who have been sexually abused have any findings at the time of medical examination. This is partially due to the nature of the sexual contact, and partially related to the fact that more long-standing sexual abuse, particularly when the abuser is very familiar to the child, rarely declares itself within a sufficiently short time of the abuse to allow for medical findings to remain. Forensic evidence which would link the abuse to the perpetrator is even rarer. (1988: 100)

There has been a significant literature on the symptomology of sexual abuse and numerous lists identifying signs and symptoms relating to it. (See for example, Glaser and Frosh, 1988; Brown et al., 1987.) Whilst a familiarity with them is useful, these lists may in themselves create difficulties for the practitioner. Salter emphasizes that

because children frequently do not reveal abuse, several authors have suggested 'laundry lists' of behaviour or symptoms thought to indicate abuse in the absence of a verbal report. However such lists are generally too non-specific to differentiate sexual abuse from other clinical problems. (1988: 233)

Jones and McQuiston note that although

a change in behaviour is common when a child has been sexually abused, in general, children tend to respond to specific stresses in non-specific ways behaviourally. This is the case in sexual abuse too. The most common behavioural consequences in the victim are neurotic disorders or disturbances of conduct that may be of a relatively non-specific nature. (1988: 3)

However, whilst sexual abuse cannot be inferred from signs and symptoms alone, there are certain indicators which seem to be more strongly associated with sexual abuse than others. Particular kinds of sexualized behaviour, either in response to other children or adults as discussed below, or the child acting alone, such as in compulsive public masturbation, seem to be highly indicative of an abusive experience.

Salter comments that

non abused children do not typically force other children to engage in sexual activity. A child who is holding down, threatening or physically harming or tying another child whilst engaging in sexual behaviour is likely to have been sexually abused themselves. (1988: 233)

She also notes as strong indicators somatic symptoms with a sexual content, physical signs, paternal jealousy, running away from home and prostitution. Other behaviours, particularly when present in an extreme form do seem to be characteristically linked with sexual abuse. Pervasive sleep and eating disorders seem particularly common. They may continue well into adulthood, long after the abuse has stopped, unless the underlying emotional causes are attended to.

Recognition and understanding of the possible indicators of child sexual abuse make an important contribution to the therapist's knowledge base and places the therapist in a better position to engage in a meaningful therapeutic relationship with the child. Where the therapist is aware at the outset that the child has been sexually abused, there are a number of specific issues to think about when planning the therapeutic session. We shall now turn to these issues.

SPECIFIC ISSUES AT THE PLANNING STAGE – THERAPY FOR ALL?

Whether all sexually abused children should be offered some therapeutic intervention and how helpful it might be is still an area of debate. This is particularly due to the difficulties posed by research and evaluation of the outcomes of therapy. Gomes-Schwartz et al. state that

most of the published data on the long-term adverse effects of sexual abuse have been derived from samples of victims who received no treatment during childhood. ... In contrast all the children in this study received some degree of therapeutic intervention, usually quite soon after the revelation of sexual abuse ... one might speculate that the relatively low rates of significant psychiatric disturbance in these children were attributable to their having received therapy ... at this time however judgement must be reserved as there is no way to test out our hypothesis. It is not possible to state with any certainty that children who do not receive services are worse in the short or long run than those who are treated, and research designs that permit such comparison are either unfeasible or unethical. (1990: 150–152)

In our view it is helpful to offer each child who has experienced sexual abuse a short sequence of non-directive play therapy sessions, with the option to continue if the child so wishes. The non-directive approach, with its emphasis on the child's choice and control of issues and of the pace of his therapy is, we feel, a very effective and non-intrusive way of working with a sexually abused child.

THE CHILD'S VIEW OF THERAPY

The sexually abused child may have a heightened awareness and sensitivity to the therapeutic sessions. These feelings need to be acknowledged by the therapist and explored with the child. Initial issues may include how the child explains the sessions to his peer group and others, and whether he feels stigmatized by therapy. These problems need to be addressed if they are not to undermine any benefit the child might derive from therapy. The therapist should also be aware that the sexually abused child may feel at the outset that therapy and the abusive situation have features in common. Haugaard and Reppucci state that

clinicians may tell children that they have a special relationship in which what they say and do will remain confidential. To a young child this may appear to be the same sort of secret relationship fostered and insisted on by the abuser. (1988: 238)

In the non-directive approach, whilst the therapist talks to the child in terms of the privacy and confidentiality offered by the therapeutic session, confidentiality cannot be absolute. The child is offered privacy but he is also told that he is free to leave the session when he chooses and free to discuss the content of the session with whomever he chooses.

The confidentiality offered to the child by the therapist is constrained by certain limits. For example, a disclosure of abuse or re-abuse by a child in a session would need to be shared with those professionals involved in child protection. This should be clear to both the child and the therapist, for the therapist has a responsibility not only to the child she sees in therapy but to other children/adolescents who may be currently being abused by the same perpetrator. The way in which issues surrounding confidentiality are explored, the timing of the discussion and the age and understanding of the child must all be considerations. The inability to offer complete confidentiality will inevitably have some effect on the quality and depth of the relationship which can be established with the child. However, it also provides a complete contrast to the emphasis on secrecy experienced within the abusive relationship.

Haugaard and Reppucci also point out that "therapy may include a good deal of sexually oriented play or discussions of sexual matters, and such play or discussion may also have occurred with the abuser" (1988: 238). In non-directive play therapy it is the child who leads rather than the therapist, and as a result the child has more control over the play materials used during the sessions. He is therefore less likely to be overwhelmed by feelings and play associated with the abuse than he might be in a more structured and directive approach.

Nevertheless the therapist does need to be aware that some of the play materials may have a specific and sexual meaning for the child. For example, Angela, eight years, responded to a toy camera in the play therapy room by taking off her pants and lying on the floor with her legs spread wide apart. The child, it was subsequently discovered, had been subjected to sexual abuse involving pornography.

THE REFERRAL STAGE

The therapist needs to have an understanding and awareness of the professional intervention in the child's life prior to referral for therapy. The sexually abused child is likely to have been involved in a validation interview which may have been recorded, and probably a medical examination. Consequently he may enter therapy either very resistant to it, or conversely too open to it, feeling that he has no choice but to repeat the abusive experiences in detail to the therapist. In non-directive therapy however the child has the opportunity to place the sexual abuse in the context of his life, rather than to be prescribed or defined by it. There are many issues the child will choose to explore in the therapeutic sessions which could not possibly have been addressed during the validation interview, with its focus on fact and information gathering (see chapter 7).

TIMING

The timing of the therapy is an important factor affecting both the accessibility of the child's feelings in relation to the abuse and the extent to which he will have developed entrenched coping mechanisms to deal with the experience. If referral to therapy takes place before civil and criminal proceedings, the permission of the court should be sought before therapy commences. In these circumstances the sessions need to be completely documented, and taped where appropriate, as well as ensuring the therapist does not spend additional, unaccounted time with the child outside of the therapeutic sessions. Only in this way can allegations of contamination of the child's evidence by the therapist effectively be countered. Where audio/videotapes are made of therapeutic sessions, it should be assumed that these tapes will be called as evidence in any subsequent court proceedings. These recordings must be intact, rather than edited versions of sessions in order to be used as complete records of therapeutic interventions. Careful thought needs to be given to audio/video recording of therapy sessions, particularly when the child may have been involved in pornography. Even though recordings provide needed safeguards for possible evidence and/or allegations its use may well shift the child's focus from his inner world to concerns and anxieties created by the recording of the therapy session itself.

With the increasing knowledge of the possible long-term damaging consequences to mental health from child sexual abuse there is an increased likelihood that therapeutic help will be sought for an abused child during the investigative stage. This is not, however, always the case, and where the child or adolescent seems to be coping well enough, the view may well be that it will be less damaging to leave things alone.

Nina, for example, waited two-and-a-half-years before a referral for therapy was made. She appeared to be a quiet, withdrawn child, who cried frequently and had frightening nightmares. Nina had been sexually assaulted by an older cousin who had lived with the family. He had been removed following the abuse and she had not seen him since. The offences had not been discussed, explored or, indeed, even mentioned since the investigation and medical examination had been completed. The difficulties created by delaying therapy are evident. The child's experiences will have become less accessible and the feelings of confusion and shame surrounding the incidents exacerbated by the subsequent lengthy silence of family and others.

Although there may be similarities in the way in which the child who is still in crisis and the child who has developed mechanisms to deal with their feelings work through their emotions, the former is likely to have an immediacy and a directness which is absent in the latter. It is clearly going to be more threatening to the child to be asked to give up coping mechanisms which have served, however imperfectly, to help him survive the past months or years.

Undoubtedly a number of children would benefit from being able to return to non-directive therapy at a later stage in their development, for example puberty or pregnancy. In these transition periods, many of the issues surrounding the abusive experience may re-emerge, despite the child now living in a secure, consistent and loving environment.

Penny, seventeen years old, for instance, began to look back on the sexual abuse she had been subjected to during her childhood. She became increasingly burdened by a sense of guilt and responsibility for not ending the abuse earlier, feelings which had not been in evidence when she had disclosed the abuse.

Penny stated

to start with I didn't know. But when I did I could easily have stopped it long before I did. I know society says I was the victim. But in the same respect so is my uncle. And he's the only one who got punished, so now I have to punish myself.

DISTANCE

The physical distance between the therapist and child always merits consideration. This is particularly true for the sexually abused child. The child has already experienced an intrusion on his personal space, privacy and perhaps body, by the perpetrator. In non-directive therapy the child maintains the control over distance between himself and the therapist. The need to decide on where to place himself in the room in relation to the therapist may itself highlight some of the difficulties the child is facing. He may find it impossible to decide, or wish to please or seek to establish the beginnings of a relationship primarily through touch. The possibility of the child exhibiting sexualized behaviour is an important issue both within therapy and a personal issue for the therapist herself. We shall return to consider this in more depth in later parts of the chapter.

THE USE OF ANATOMICALLY CORRECT DOLLS

The child may find it helpful to use the anatomically correct dolls to re-enact concretely the abusive experience and associated feelings. However, unless the therapist is clear from the outset that the child has been sexually abused, it seems unnecessary and potentially damaging to introduce the dolls routinely. The dolls' role in therapy is an open question; whether the dolls are in themselves potentially disturbing and/or sexualizing is unresolved. The use the child has made of the dolls, if any, during the validation interview may give some indication as to their usefulness during subsequent therapy sessions. Their use will always require careful consideration; the dolls are so specialized that they will not have been seen by the child outside a professional setting. (See also chapter 7. section 3.)

ISSUES AND THEMES EMERGING IN THERAPY

Although, as we indicated earlier, the child who has been sexually abused may experience difficulties in common with an emotionally damaged child, certain themes and issues are particularly characteristic of therapy with the sexually abused child.

The form and intensity of these themes, and indeed whether they appear at all, will depend on the emotional impact which the abuse has had on the child. This may vary greatly, depending for example on the context in which it took place, the age of the child, the relationship with the abuser, the availability of other loving relationships, and the distance in time between the occurrence of the abuse and the time of the referral. Glaser and Frosh point out that there are

differences between those children who were abused when young but whose abuse was terminated by early intervention, and those who continue to be abused over many years. Other differences arise in relation to the emotional proximity of the abuser to the child, the mother and the family and especially to the degree of secrecy and coercion associated with the abuse. Secrecy is particularly harmful, but the effects of coercion are more complex; coercion will increase a child's fear and sense of helplessness but sometimes reduces her sense of guilt. (1988: 117)

FEELINGS EXPRESSED OR EXPERIENCED

The feelings experienced by the sexually abused child or adolescent and likely to be expressed during therapy have been raised to some degree earlier in this chapter. They are predominantly negative in character. Feelings of anxiety, fear, vulnerability, helplessness, hopelessness, guilt, shame, anger, resentment and depression are familiar and well documented in the literature (Sgroi, 1989). These feelings if left unresolved may lead to a distorted perception of self, poor self-esteem and may continue into adulthood.

Those feelings associated with the abuse that seemed more positive at the time, for example, experiencing the relationship as offering emotional support, affection and love, may create serious difficulties for the child subsequently, either leading to increased self-blame and guilt, particularly if the offender received a custodial sentence, or to interference with future relationships. The sexual abuse frequently engenders feelings of ambivalence and confusion towards the perpetrator and the non-protective carer. The sexual abuse often takes place in the context of what is presented as a loving relationship. The abuser may be a source, sometimes the only source of affection for the child. The child may, through extra privileges or attention, benefit from being sexually available; where the child experiences physical pleasure during the abuse he may feel additional guilt at his enjoyment.

This dissonance between mental distaste for the experience and physical arousal may be particularly threatening to the child. Where sexual arousal is experienced by a child or adolescent who has not yet established, or is struggling to integrate, sexual feelings within their sense of self, it is unsurprising that sexual abuse gives rise to acute feelings of ambivalence and guilty confusion. The dilemma is heightened for boys, who may resolve their confusion and fears of homosexuality by identification with their abuser (Benton, 1991).

The non-directive approach is well suited to working with the child's ambivalent feelings, since the therapist makes no assumptions about what the child will be feeling and is concerned to acknowledge and help the child to make sense of his ambivalence. This clarification and exploration of uncertain feelings is illustrated in the following play sequence with a sexually abused child. In the sequence the therapist reflects back the child's feelings, as well as using her own feelings of repulsion and being dominated, in a congruent and therapeutic way. The therapist enables the child, then, to distinguish his own feelings, the feelings of the abuser, and the feelings of both abuser and child interacting together, in the less threatening environment of the play therapy room. In addition, the child is less threatened because he is himself taking the dominant role of the abuser.

William, age six, in an excited state, made a large penis out of playdough and thrust the object with both hands towards the therapist's mouth.

> **William:** You like it.
>
> **Therapist:** You want me to like it. But I don't like it.
>
> **William:** [becoming insistent] You do like it.
>
> **Therapist:** You're telling me that I have to like it, but I don't like it.

Role taking play in which the child assigns the therapist the role of the child while he himself takes the adult role has been discussed in chapter 2. By reversing roles the child is able to differentiate his own and the adult's emotions more clearly and consider both perspectives at once.

The child's feelings of ambivalence and confusion may relate to other significant family members whether or not they have had direct knowledge of or a role in the abusive experience. Jenny, in the following extract from a non-directive play therapy session, began to explore the terrifying nightmares she had been having, within the security of the therapeutic relationship.

Jenny chose to paint the nightmare which threatened her most. The therapist in her acceptance of the child's fearful and mistrustful feelings of her mother enabled the child to explore what it was about her mother and their relationship which created such anxiety. The mother's changed appearance in the painting and nightmare reflected the child's fear that her mother would turn against her, as she had turned against her cousin and brother following the sexual abuse – for which Jenny felt in some way responsible. She also missed her cousin, and had affectionate feelings for him, but was not permitted to speak about these at home.

Jenny painted her mother's face. The eyes in the face were empty, white, but not expressionless; they appeared distant and cruel.

> **Jenny:** They [her eyes] were really frightening ... and then she [mother] came to me and threw me down on the floor, hit me across the head and kicked me.
>
> **Therapist** Knew it was mum, but some things were so different – her eyes, white ... just white and staring ... and seeing them almost more frightening than being hurt.

Jenny tore the painting up when she had completed it. By having something concrete to destroy, to have control over, she could begin to control her fear.

> **Therapist:** And tearing it up, a way to get rid of it. Those eyes not looking at you anymore, can't frighten you anymore.

The following account of another child's confused feelings towards his abusing carer is from the first session with James, a six-year-old placed in foster care a year earlier following the death of an older (female) cousin. She had brought him up from the age of two years, after his mother had rejected him. It illustrates the difficulty which a child has in coming to terms with the contradictory feelings of grief at the loss of his most significant relationship, the pleasure, confusion and anger over the abuse, and his sexualized responses to it.

Although the therapist appears to say little it is worth noting that an assessment undertaken shortly after the boy's placement, which focused in particular on work with the anatomically correct dolls, had concluded that this child had not been sexually abused.

James, age six, looked sad. He talked about the death of his cousin, wishing that she was still alive. He sat on the floor very close to the therapist. In a hesitant manner he said, "I could tell you a lot about her, like a lot of books I've been keeping locked in a trunk. Maybe I might tell you about the first chapter." He talked about living with his cousin. "We always slept together. She'd tell me to put my head on her (nervous smile) titties." He continued in a resigned voice, "She'd tell me to suck them. Then she'd tell me to lay on top of her. She'd hold me between her legs, you know." The boy turned his head away his face flushed with shame, "You don't want to hear all of the first chapter do you?" he whispered.

He described his cousin's regular abuse of him, including anal digital penetration and oral intercourse. As he described some of his experiences, he became angry. "I was racing my car, crashing it against the front of the bed. I wished it would bounce back and crash into her head. She said if anyone found out, we couldn't do it anymore and I'd be taken away for good." Even fully dressed, it became obvious that he was also sexually aroused as he talked.

This demonstrates a range of feelings that the child was experiencing, including ambivalence towards his abuser. It also shows how important it is for the therapist not to impose her own feelings about what has occurred on the child. As Glaser and Frosh point out: "Ambivalent feelings of anger and fondness for the abuser are not easily expressed in a context which strongly disapproves of the abuser and the abuse." (1988: 117)

Loss, evident here, is also a strong theme for children and adolescents who have experienced sexual abuse. Loss in terms of childhood innocence, due to the sexualization of relationships, and loss of control over body, feelings, choice and privacy. Loss may well extend to loss of contact with the abuser, for example, if the abuser receives a custodial sentence. Equally it may result in loss of other family members if moved to an alternative placement, and loss in many instances of school, friends and familiar environment.

SEXUALIZED BEHAVIOUR

While the exploration of the child's feelings takes a central place in therapy, the child's behaviour may also demonstrate to the therapist the way in which the child has come to terms with the sexual abuse, and the conflict created by it.

Children who have been sexually abused, particularly over a long period of time, may inadvertently behave towards others in ways that are seen as seductive. Where the abuse has taken place within the context of a loving relationship, they may be unable to distinguish between sexual and non-sexual ways of expressing love and affection.

These children may wish to recreate their sexual experiences within the therapeutic relationship. Sometimes the child may re-enact part of the abusive experience in an attempt to get in touch with it, and to come to terms with the trauma, by playing it out in the therapeutic setting. In non-directive play therapy the child retains control over the outcome of his re-enactment in addition to having the support and acceptance of the therapist.

Lucy, age ten, in her use of clay during a play therapy session began to explore her predominantly, and at times disabling, feelings of fear in relation to her father who had abused her. In the therapist's reflection of her actions and the feelings associated with them, Lucy was able to begin to come to terms with this fear of her father.

Lucy began to shape the clay into a man's head.

> **Therapist:** Beginning to take shape now.

> **Lucy:** [nodding, concentrating, serious] Yes, this is going to be him.

> **Therapist:** You're sure who it will be.

> **Lucy:** It's him, it's dad.

> **Therapist:** Creating dad, here in this room.

His head was given a long, thick, almost erect nose. Lucy pulled at this, rubbed it, smoothed it, shaped it until its shape and feeling satisfied her, then she wrenched it off.

> **Therapist:** Tearing that part of him off, getting rid of it, he can't have that part now ... angry with that part of him ... all of him.

Lucy, nodding, was already re-creating the head shape, repeating the process of re-forming and mutilating it a number of times. Finally she shaped the head again, this time the nose was of normal size and appearance. She turned urgently to the clay again and forming a bowl shaped receptacle with it, punched her fist into it hard.

> **Therapist:** Forcing it in.

She found a toy with a round wooden handle and thrust this into the clay repeatedly. Her eyes became unfocused, her breathing heavier.

> **Therapist:** In again and again, building up. You're doing it, pushing it in again and again, almost that you can't stop.

Lucy reached a climax of activity and stopped. The clay was left, the child began to relax.

> **Therapist:** And once you had started, no way to stop, on and on until it was over, and a relief it's over.

In her symbolic mutilation and hence control over her father's nose (penis), she experienced the feelings of being omnipotent, the controller of her father, in fact his abuser. With the re-working of this theme a number of times during the session she began to gain mastery over her feelings and to resolve the conflict which had been engendered in her. Towards the end of this session she was able to reform her father's head into a more 'normal' shape and to be able to tolerate a less fearful, punitive and angry feeling towards him. She again took the role of activist and abuser in her 'penetration' of the clay shape during which she re-experienced the physical sensation of orgasm alongside a feeling that nothing could stop this action once it began. Lucy was not able to verbalize her feelings; however this powerful re-enactment, and the therapist's ability to reflect the symbolic play and her deeper feelings associated with it, enabled her to begin to be able to integrate her experiences into her current functioning and to come to terms with them.

On other occasions the child's sexualized behaviour may reflect his pre-dominant need for affection; his sexualized advance is his attempt to gain that affection. The child may be trying to differentiate between acceptable and unacceptable behaviour, or he may have become sexually aroused and wish to draw the therapist into the experience. Depending therefore on the purpose the sexualized behaviour has for the child within the session, the therapeutic task may be, in reflecting on the behaviour, to help the child draw appropriate boundaries and to learn about acceptable touching and contact. The therapist's response enables the child to explore different and more acceptable ways of meeting his needs, without inducing further guilt. It allows the child, as Glaser and Frosh suggest, "to retain a concept of sexuality as enjoyable and permissible, albeit in the appropriate context". (1988: 116)

SELF-MUTILATION

The child may internalize his angry and aggressive feelings rather than channel them toward the abuser or non-protective parent. This may be because of fear of further assaults, rejection or abandonment. These internalized angry feelings may result in the child's self-mutilation.

Self-mutilation seems most likely to occur with those children who have experienced a long-standing, incestuous relationship where there have been feelings of attachment to or identification with the abuser, some pleasure associated with the experience, and a commensurate feeling of guilt and self blame at enjoying it, or allowing it to continue. Where the child has inadvertently or deliberately disclosed the abuse and in doing so 'betrayed' the secret and the abuser, the feelings may be predominantly those of self-punishment and blame. Also present may be a sense of defilement, with self-mutilation the outward expression of inward disgust for the child's body.

As Anderson states:

feeling depressed and guilty ... they sought to damage their bodies, which they saw as sullied, or to render their bodies less attractive and therefore less tempting, or they sought to blot out the memory of pleasure with self-inflicted pain. (quoted in Haugaard and Reppucci, 1988: 69)

In the following excerpt from a play therapy session Amy, age twelve, began to explore, in response to the therapist's reflections, some of the feelings associated with her self-mutilation which had become very disfiguring. As Amy painted, she stopped and wrote on her painting, "I can love other people. I don't love myself."

> **Therapist:** Feeling different from other people. They can be loved.
>
> **Amy:** I'm ugly and dirty – that's how I am.
>
> **Therapist:** Ugly and dirty and not lovable.
>
> **Amy:** I don't know why I pull at my face. I'm not a nice person. Inside I'm messy and disgusting.
>
> **Therapist:** You really don't like what's inside.
>
> **Amy:** When I'd been to see my sisters at Mum's I wanted to tear at my face, when I got back to [foster mother's] . . . she really let me have it when I did that.

She paused, then said sadly and wistfully, "and I don't know why I do it."

Exploring this the therapist put the two things alongside one another. Amy began the session with an awareness of her feelings of dirtiness and ugliness in relation to herself. The therapist, in placing the child's feelings alongside the self-mutilating behaviour, gave the child the opportunity to begin to link the two.

> **Therapist:** Feelings inside messy and raw and wanting to tear at your face . . . face feeling a bit raw too.

The self-mutilation stopped after three or four sessions of Amy's exploration of her feelings and the conflicts they resulted in for her.

Another example is Gail, an adolescent, who begins to explore her self-mutilation in the following extract from one, of many, therapy sessions.

> [Gail pulled up her sleeves to reveal the most recent cuts on her arms . . .]
>
> **Gail:** I do it when I'm angry.
>
> **Therapist:** And in some ways it helps with the angry feelings.
>
> **Gail:** When I really want to lose my temper.

Therapist: Cut yourself – instead of losing control of your temper.

Gail: I hate that. I hate being so angry ... and then I start to feel down because I'm so angry.

Therapist: Worse feeling your temper ... you're feeling out of control ... brings you down!

Gail: hate myself for feeling like it, and so I start to cut myself. When I'm angry, I cut away ... it's better to cut myself than hurt someone else.

Therapist: While you're hurting yourself you're not hurting anyone else.

Gail: I get really angry with my dad [her abuser] that's when I cut.

Therapist: Like the anger's turned away from your dad towards you.

Gail: I want to be angry with him but I can't. Something stopping it. [looking and sounding frightened] I'm frightened what will happen. [angrily] They [the parents] never really wanted me. I've always felt on the outside.

Therapist: Sort of pushed out by them.

Gail: And I'd like to belong.

Therapist: Really need that, feeling someone, somewhere for you.

Gail: Now my heart says stay, but my head tells me to move on.

Therapist: Heart and head telling you different things, stay and go, like they're competing.

Gail: [wearily] And my head wins.

Therapist: Head wins over the feelings of wanting to stay.

[Gail talked of her most recent hospital admission, when she had cut her wrists again.]

Gail: [brightening up] I don't mind. I know the ropes.

Therapist: Familiar, almost like going home.

> **Gail:** [smiling] The nurses are really nice to me, they're really pleased to see me.
>
> **Therapist:** You have a real place there, they like you to be there.
>
> **Gail:** I feel part of something.
>
> **Therapist:** Almost like your family.

This sequence began with her exploration of angry feelings resulting in the self-mutilation. It then moved on to a deeper feeling of loss of temper and its association with loss of control, together with Gail's fear of being out of control now. This was reminiscent for her of the abusive experience when she had not had control and her father's apparent loss of control. During this exploration another feeling associated with the self-mutilation was differentiated. This concerned her very profound feelings of rejection and abandonment by her mother, and having no safe place where she belonged. Gail then was able to take a look at her self-mutilation as a route into the safety and security of the hospital environment; the only place she felt she really belonged and where she had a right to be.

Peter identified the rather different purpose that the self-mutilation had for him. He retained fearful and angry feelings towards his father with whom he identified, and ambivalent feelings towards his mother who had not cared for and protected him. In this sequence he is able to acknowledge his positive feelings towards his mother and stepfather and his hitherto unexpressed desperate need for them.

> Peter proudly held up his arms on which he had tattooed his mother's and stepfather's names.
>
> **Therapist:** Your mum and step-dad's names in ink ... always there on your arms.
>
> **Peter:** Yes, because they'll be with me for ever.

The pain inflicted during the self-mutilation may represent the child's attempt to re-experience the physical self, where the method of coping with the sexual abuse has been to detach the mind from what the body is experiencing. Then self-mutilaton may be a means of reintegrating this physical and mental activity. We shall consider this more fully under the heading of dissociation.

Although, therefore, in general self-mutilation may be readily identified as the expression of guilt and the need for self-punishment, it is important to remain alert to the specific meaning the behaviour has for the particular child. Whether it is an expression of anger (thwarted) at the abuser; self-blame for having experienced some physical pleasure during the abuse, or for having disclosed it; a wish to defile an already defiled body; a means of distracting oneself, through inflicting physical pain, from the inward psychic pain; or a wish to get in touch with physical sensation from which one has become detached. During adolescence, and its associated stronger sexual urges, these may become linked to the sexual abuse and result in the young person mutilating breasts and/or genital area. When the scarring from self-mutilation is extensive, it serves as a constant reminder to the child of the abusive experience. Not least, it signifies to the outside world that the child is hurting and is in need of help.

DISSOCIATIVE REACTIONS

Dissociative reactions, such as amnesia and out of body responses during the abuse, are the child's psychological defence against a seriously traumatizing experience from which he cannot physically escape. Where the need to separate the sexual abuse from the rest of the child's life is very strong, the denial may involve the almost total separation of self which has experienced the abuse from the self which functions in the everyday world.

For a better understanding of the process of this splitting of experience from self, we return to Piaget's view that all experience involves a person's total reaction. Piaget in discussing the origins of intelligence in infants' notes that "almost since birth ... there is 'behaviour' in the sense of the individual's total reaction and not a setting in motion of particular or local automatizations only interrelated from within." (1952: 24) In order to integrate his experience the child must engage in internal constructive activity. Where the experience has been that of sexual abuse, to integrate this abuse into other predominantly motor schemas the child must engage in an active, constructive activity and relate it to his current functioning. Yet a conflict exists for the child, for in the experience of sexual abuse the child's body is used in an abnormal way by the abuser. His body is used in an intimate way that is disapproved of by society, but may evoke certain pleasurable sensations in the child. A conflict exists, then, in the child's desire for action (motor level schemas). The child experiences a conflict between obedience to the abuser and escape from the abuse. In real life the only solutions to this conflict are submission, escape or co-operation. (Of course, the child may not necessarily have conscious awareness of possible solutions to his conflict.)

Submission and co-operation may be indistinguishable for the sexually abused child. The abuser will often use persuasion to gain the child's co-operation. He may also tell the child that the experience is good, that the child is special to him, and that the child is enjoying it. The child may consciously assume he is co-operating rather than submitting, because of his immature thought processes and his malleability. At another level, however, he may be aware of his conflicting feelings or consciously feel guilty about the experience. These conflicts of feeling are difficult to integrate into his developing affective schemas. This will especially be the case when the abuser is also a person within the family where relatively permanent affective schemas will have been developed by the child in relation to family members (for example, love, jealousy).

A conflict also exists for the child on a bodily level. The elementary motor schemas developed by the child in relation to his own body – for example, sucking as a baby, excretion, use of his hands for exploration and manipulation – will be distorted by the sexual abuse. Because it always involves parts of the child's body, and especially if it involves a family member and intimate parts of his body as well, the abuse will affect relatively permanent and basic motor and affective schemas. As the sexual acts are so intimately associated with the core of the child's personality (ego) then their relation to the ego may be repressed by the abused child. The child may feel dirty and worthless, and even if these feelings are openly acknowledged by him, he may not be able to integrate the motor activities involved in the abuse into his existing motor schemas. Indeed, where integration does take place, this is likely to have more serious implications for the child because the distortion is internalized and less accessible to therapeutic help. Where the child dissociates his mind from his bodily experiences in order to cope with the abuse, re-enactment in therapy will help him to reintegrate his traumatic experiences into healthier schemas.

In non-directive play therapy the child can work through, at his own pace if and when he chooses to do so, the dissociation of body parts, for example in the use of his hands or his mouth, which may have been involved in the abuse (say, during oral intercourse) within the permissive environment of the therapeutic session. Play activity is an important aspect of this therapeutic involvement. The sexual abuse and its aftermath create for the child inescapable conflicts in reality. In play, however, these conflicts can be creatively worked on to integrate them into the ego at an acceptable level. The play activity can remain on a symbolic level. Examples already noted are when the child made a penis out of playdough, or the child repeatedly penetrated the clay with hand and then object. The child can safely use, within the therapeutic session, some areas of his body that have been involved in the sexual abuse, for instance, his hands or mouth, since it is socially acceptable to expose them. The child clearly cannot deal directly with other more intimate parts of his body that may have been involved in the abuse, but can do so symbolically as noted above.

Children play symbolically on different levels. At one extreme are symbols used in play that involve permanent and basic affective and motor schemas. At this extreme, as we have illustrated, symbolic play makes use of personal schemas embodying "matters of intimate, permanent concerns, of secret and inexpressible desires". (Piaget, 1962: 175) At the other end of the continuum are objective schemas related to activities without hidden extra meanings. Piaget gives an example of a child pretending he is a steeple. "He is expressing what interests him in the widest sense of the word and there is certainly assimilation of reality to the ego. But these interests are only temporary." (1962: 175)

The child attempting through dissociation to escape the conflicts which are associated with his sexual abuse, may play them out symbolically in non-directive play therapy. Whilst the therapist should have the ability to talk about the child's symbolic play in order to make the play more conscious for the child, the child himself does not necessarily need to talk about it. The child can work through the conflicts symbolically and in this way re-integrate them in a healthy way. For other children verbalization does seem to be a necessary therapeutic experience. An older child, Michelle, in the following extract, was able to verbalize her dissociative experiences.

[Michelle described how she would 'leave her body' during the abuse].

Michelle: It was like I could leave what was happening.

Therapist: Found a way to get away.

Michelle: Not my body. I couldn't get that away but – you'll think I'm mad. I was up on the ceiling, looking down.

Therapist: Like the part of you that hurts and feels could leave and look down ... almost as if what was happening down there was unreal.

Michelle: That's it – I'd look down, and it was like a dream, no noise, it didn't hurt, it was just happening.

Therapist: Watching, but it didn't feel real, almost like it wasn't happening to you.

Michelle: It was me. I knew it was me, but it was alright.

Therapist: It was happening, you couldn't stop it happening, but you could manage it like this.

Michelle said these 'out of body' experiences had happened a number of times. The first time had been during a particularly violent assault. Later it had happened when she had heard her abuser's footsteps coming up the stairs. More recently it had happened when she was being interviewed by a police officer and social worker following her disclosure of the abuse.

During her sessions Michelle was able to reflect on these experiences when she 'left' her body. She explored how it had begun, the purpose it had served for her – an escape route when she felt all others were closed – and the triggers for it. It was de-mystified for her. Whilst it had not frightened her during the abusive assaults, the fact that it had continued to happen when the abuse stopped made Michelle feel out of control, frightened and at times that she was going mad.

Another response of adults in traumatic situations is amnesia. It seems more likely when working with children and adolescents that there will be a less extreme form of denial of the experience than amnesia. For instance some children minimize the impact of the abuse: "it wasn't really important ... it didn't really matter to me." Nevertheless, amnesia or the 'forgetting' of the abusive experience does occur. Since therapy works all the time on the edge of the conscious mind, it is likely that, as described earlier, much therapy will involve the bringing into conscious awareness aspects of the sexual experience of which the child has been previously unaware. For example, Betty gradually came to face her fear of 'the black hole' which she sensed at some level contained other disturbing experiences.

> **Betty:** It's funny. I can't remember anything about being little.

> **Therapist:** Those early years seem lost.

> **Betty:** I just can't remember.

> **Therapist:** Just nothing at all ... and it troubles you.

> **Betty:** A big black hole. [whispered]

> **Therapist:** And it might be frightening.

> **Betty:** I daren't look into it ... something happened to me ... I don't know what. I think something else awful happened to me, worse, I can't remember but I feel that it did.

She was then able to bring into consciousness not only the memory of her earlier abusive experiences but also a recapturing of happier childhood days which had previously been lost to her.

As an adult Fraser (1989) in her moving autobiographical account of being abused by her father throughout her middle childhood, describes how she repressed all conscious awareness of the abuse, and developed into a lively, attractive and successful teenager and young woman. The effort (unconscious) to sustain the repression of the knowledge of the abuse became more untenable; awareness of it gradually 'leaked' into her conscious mind and she was gradually able to assimilate and integrate these abusive experiences.

EATING AND SLEEPING DISTURBANCES

Finally, we turn to sleeping and eating disturbances, which are often most noticeable amongst sexually abused children.

Whilst anorexia and bulimia are both correlated with the possibility of sexual abuse, obesity also seems to serve a purpose for some sexually abused children. Edward, for example, felt that his weight would mean that he, as a bigger and stronger child, could better defend himself against his father's sexual advances. Tina, in contrast, hoped that by eating as little as possible she would appear more boylike and consequently be less attractive to her stepfather and that his abuse of her would stop.

Disturbances in sleep patterns are also a familiar theme for children and adolescents who have been sexually abused. Bedtime is frequently associated with the abusive experiences and becomes a time of fear rather than relaxation. Young children may become so tense and stressed at night that they are unable to sleep, older children may find ways to compensate for their lack of night time sleep.

Naomi had developed a pattern of using catnaps during the day and evening whilst her mother was at home to protect her, to mitigate the loss of sleep during the night. Despite dragging a chest of drawers across her bedroom door each night, she still remained awake for as long as possible in case her stepfather tried to assault her again.

ISSUES FOR THE THERAPIST

Feelings

The therapist also needs to think through the implications for herself, as an individual, of working with a sexually abused child. She may find what the child says or does, or the child's experiences, so shocking or overwhelming that to cope with these events the therapist herself blocks out certain feelings or themes. The therapist needs the kind of supervision which would allow her to explore the emotional impact of the work on her.

Intrusive sexual thoughts or sexual responses to the child's sexualized behaviour in therapy are often disturbing and difficult to deal with. There seem to be a number of issues of which the therapist needs to be aware. The explicit or diffused sexuality of the child may evoke, in addition to sexual feelings, a physical arousal in the therapist. It is important for the therapist to be able to acknowledge this to herself privately and to explore it subsequently in supervision with a colleague who is experienced and knowledgeable in this area of work. The therapist needs a clear understanding of acceptable boundaries within the therapeutic relationship. This is vitally important in work with the sexually abused child whose boundaries have been distorted by the abusive experience. Within supervision the therapist can explore these boundaries and additionally clarify and differentiate between her own feelings and responses and the child's. The therapist, having acknowledged her own response and feelings privately, must decide whether it is therapeutically enabling to share these with the child. Such a decision would be highly exceptional but might be felt necessary if a male therapist has become obviously physically aroused and the child has noticed or commented on this. Note that in this case, as in all other issues during non-directive play therapy, it would be the child who, either verbally or non-verbally, directed attention to the therapist's response and initiated the topic, rather than the therapist.

Gender of the therapist

Clearly in the above discussion the gender of the therapist has implications for the kind of physical arousal occurring in the therapy session. Jehu concludes that

The psychotherapy literature generally provides no unequivocal conclusions on the influence of the gender of the therapist and no clear guidelines as to the optimal client–therapist matching on the basis of this variable. (Jehu et al., 1989: 31)

As long as the advantages and disadvantages of a male or female therapist working with the child are addressed, Furniss believes that there "is no reason why women cannot work with children abused by women or men with children abused by men" (1991: 293). The child should ideally be given the choice of a male or female therapist at the outset of therapy. (See other references for a fuller discussion of the advantages and disadvantages of male or female therapists, for example Furniss, 1991.)

Potential drawbacks to having a male therapist are that he may become more easily sexually aroused, identify with a male abuser or collude with the child against the maternal figure. The advantages may be that a male therapist offers the child the different experience of a non-sexualized, safe, warm, caring relationship with a man. Obviously, this would only be helpful if the child could tolerate and manage the mistrust and fear of being alone with the male therapist. A male therapist may also be better able to deal with the child's positive feelings about a male abuser. (However, this may not always be the case: see, for example Frosh, 1987, for a counter example.)

A disadvantage of having a female therapist can be that she may more easily identify with the child and as a result be less able to allow ambivalent or pleasurable feelings about the abuser to be expressed. Additionally the child's ambivalent or hostile feelings relating to the maternal figure may be threatening for the therapist. The female therapist may also find it less easy to acknowledge her sometimes more diffused sexualized responses.

The advantages often cited for having a female therapist are that the child who has experienced sexual abuse may find it easier to talk to a female therapist, particularly if the perpetrator is male. The female therapist may also offer the child a different model to a non-protective or rejecting maternal figure.

Since however, we would in general concur with Jehu et al. in considering that there is as yet no unequivocal evidence concerning the impact of the gender of the therapist, where there is the possibility of choice, decisions in individual cases will need to be made on the basis of one's best judgement concerning the aetiology of the problem and the circumstances of the particular child.

We have in this chapter considered the particular themes and issues which emerge in therapy with the sexually abused child or adolescent. In our next and concluding chapter we focus on four specific areas of practice which the therapist will need to consider in non-directive therapy.

7

Practice Skills and Issues

REFLECTION

In his book **Client-Centred Therapy**, Rogers (1976) explores somewhat ruefully the difficulty of accurately conveying what the task of the non-directive Rogerian counsellor is. He highlights the ways in which the worker's role may be misinterpreted on the one hand by being seen as passive and disengaged, involving a "minimum of activity and of emotional reaction", and on the other hand as a cognitive process of classification of the client's problem rather than an emphatic communication of understanding:

it is hard accurately to convey to a reader the delicate attitudes involved in the therapist's work. We have learned, to our dismay, that even the transcripts of our recorded cases may give to the reader a totally erroneous notion of the sort of relationship which existed. (1976: 27–28)

We have throughout this book, given illustrative examples of the way in which the therapist may reflect an understanding of what the child is experiencing, and through this, support the child in achieving mastery over feelings of, say, conflict, loss or anger. In chapter 2, we developed a framework for understanding how the process of play enables the child through the development of different schema, to assimilate and integrate these conflicting feelings. It seems appropriate, especially in the light of Rogers's caveat (above), to focus in this section on one of the skills involved in assisting this process, namely the core skill of recognizing what the child is experiencing, and reflecting this in a non-threatening manner.

In focusing on this specific skill, we are aware of setting aside a fuller discussion of the principles underlying the process of accurate empathy. The reader is referred elsewhere for such a discussion, and a consideration of some of the research which attempts to identify the therapeutic qualities of empathy. (Mearns and Thorne, 1990; Truax and Carkhuff, 1967)

We start by addressing some of the difficulties which beginning therapists commonly experience in learning to respond appropriately to the child's communication. These include a number of responses: an over intrusiveness on the part of the therapist, which although arising from a benign wish to help and encourage the child, may actually interrupt the child's process of getting in touch with what he is feeling; attempts to move the child too rapidly by suggesting ways he could find a solution to the problem; adopting a 'good parent' role, by stimulating the child instead of following the child's lead; overly complex or repetitive responses which parrot what the child has said or done rather than responding to or picking up feelings; difficulties about using one's own feelings; and interpreting rather than reflecting feelings. After examining these problems, we consider ways in which accurate reflection enables the child to move into the exploration of deeper feelings. We also consider the therapist's need to recognize and respond appropriately to the child's defensive responses.

As Mearns and Thorne point out, it is sometimes difficult to convey by single examples what is meant by an empathic response, since empathy is a process rather than a single response (1990: 39–40). However, although each example in itself may seem over particular, the cumulative effect conveyed to the child by the therapist's responses is significant.

In the early stages of therapy, as the therapist and child familiarize themselves with each other, the therapist's responses may have a rather stilted quality and appear to be more a response to the content than to the feeling which the child is expressing. (We discuss this more fully with reference to the early stages of Helen's therapy in chapter 4.) Axline suggests at this early stage, that it may be appropriate to respond factually to questions. "Then the child can go on from there. It is often just an attempt on the part of the child to get acquainted with the therapist. What else do they have to talk about?" (1987: 98)

However, the therapist's anxiety about making contact and establishing rapport with the child may make her respond in a way which is over intrusive, and which fails to acknowledge and reflect what the child is feeling. It is important also to convey from the outset the fact that the therapy session is different from the usual adult/child communications, in that the child is free to choose what to do, and the adult will follow his lead rather than vice versa; conventional responses on the part of the therapist may make this distinction less clear.

The first session with Robin, age six, illustrates this process. This session was conducted by a beginning therapist, and was characterized by a number of attempts by her to put him at his ease, ensure that he was comfortable, and so on. For example, the therapist asked at each point at which Robin initiated a new action:

> "Do you want to take your coat off?"
>
> "Perhaps you'd like to put an apron on if you want to paint."
>
> "There are lots of things here you can play with."
>
> "Shall I roll your sleeves up for you?", and so on.

Although these were said in a gentle tone, which communicated the therapist's wish that the child should feel welcome and at home in the play session, they in fact failed to convey that the child was free to choose whether or not, in this instance, to keep his coat on, or to paint without bothering to kit himself up; nor did they accurately respond to what the child himself was feeling. (In later sessions, Robin's decision whether or not to take off his coat was an indication of his feelings about participating in the therapy; the therapist was then able to reflect his feelings, a process which was pre-empted earlier.) In the last two examples, the therapist had in fact recognized that the child was feeling some anxiety about what he would do in the play room, and some discomfort when he was trying to paint with sleves that fell down over his hands. A more empathic response, therefore, would have been one that acknowledged the therapist's recognition of these feelings, and one which also began the process of heightening the child's own awareness of what he was feeling. For example:

> "Wondering if there's anything here for you. It's sometimes hard to know what to do."
>
> "You're finding your sleeves are getting a bit in the way", followed, if the child's response indicates it is appropriate, that is, that he may want help, "I can help you roll them up if you want me to."

These responses also illustrate the difficulty which may sometimes be experienced by beginning therapists in moving from the often more familiar role of teacher or parent to that of therapist. Many adults are accustomed in their relationships with children to taking care of them (for example, seeing they are comfortable, or suitably dressed as in the examples above) or providing direction or stimulation so that the child will learn from what he is doing. Since these responses are all entirely appropriate for the good teacher or parent, it is often quite demanding to unlearn them in the therapy session. It may be difficult to resist encouraging the child by praising him for something he has drawn or made. But doing so in fact gives a different, and in this context, inappropriate message, because it reflects the content of what the child is doing and suggests there is a standard to be achieved and skills to be learned. (It may also convey, by implication, that some activities are less acceptable, or that the child could incur blame as well as praise.) In the following example, the child has been constructing figures in playdough. The therapist, impressed by the child's concentrated efforts, is eager to help him complete the construction and finds herself in a teaching or parental role:

>**Child:** I don't know what to do about the nose.

>**Therapist:** If you rolled the playdough in your hands, you could make a nose to stick on the face. That would suit it.

Note that we would distinguish between the above intervention, which is directed at helping the child move forward on a cognitive level, and the following one where the therapist responds empathetically to the child's feeling of frustration at what he experiences as the inadequacy of his painting:

>**Child:** A rainbow in the middle of nowhere. All that space and only one thing in it.

>**Therapist:** You're not happy with the picture you've drawn.

>**Child:** There's nowt there.

>**Therapist:** Feel it could be better.

>**Child:** Yeah.

>**Therapist:** Want to make it better. [The child hesitates] Not sure you can.

Another common difficulty is that in an effort to reflect rather than, say, interpret or direct, the therapist either says little or nothing, or repeats what the child has said. This may occur when the therapist is unfamiliar with the child, and is uncertain about the meaning of the child's play; it also often reflects the therapist's anxiety about the actual technique, which may in fact block her empathic response, or make her feel that anything she adds will be directive. In this example, the therapist's responses add nothing to what the child is experiencing and the latter may be becoming impatient:

>**Child:** Look, I've made a circle of dough.

>**Therapist:** You've made a circle, haven't you?

>**Child:** I can make it bigger like this.

>**Therapist:** You can make it bigger. [The child hesitates] Not sure you
>can.

>**Therapist:** You can make it bigger. [The therapist might have commented on the child's evident pleasure, for example.]

Child: I've broken it.

Therapist: It's broken.

It is also important, in working with children, to keep responses brief; when the therapist is simultaneously aware of a number of a child's feelings, it may be hard not to get too wordy. In the following sequence, the therapist is trying to acknowledge the child's feelings (about not having enough), her awareness that the child may feel she is withholding things, and her sense of being rather ungenerous at not giving, while at the same time setting a clear limit. The result is too complicated for the child to follow:

Child: Can I take it? I'd bring it back. No one would know.

Therapist: Feels as if, if no one knows then it's all right. Makes me feel mean, saying no, because it seems quite a little thing. And it's hard for you to share, not have things which are for the other children as well. You feel as if I really ought to let you.

Child: Can I? [He is not clear, and perhaps feels the therapist is weakening]

Therapist: I can't let you have it. The toys are for you and other children to use here. [The therapist finally sets the limit, clearly, and Robin moves on to drink deeply from a bottle of water]

The therapist may also, as in the earlier example with playdough, respond to cognitive material at a cogitive level because of her own preoccupation with the content, and in doing so fail to identify the emotion which lies beneath the child's verbal statement. In the following extract from another therapist's session with a disturbed eleven-year-old boy, she is preoccupied by a wish to ensure that the child remains in therapy: this intrudes on her ability to 'hear' the emotional tone of what is being communicated, and her response temporarily draws the child away from his feelings to thinking about the process of receiving help.

Henry: What good will it do to tell you about it? I don't understand.

Therapist: You mean, talking won't help?

Henry: Yes. What good will it do?

Therapist: Sometimes people feel better about things after talking them over. [When the therapist falls into the trap of answering an emotional question as if it were a mere request for information it leads to difficulties.]

Henry: Yes, but what good will it do to feel better about things if they still go on?

Therapist: Sometimes boys and girls can understand the way they really feel about things and it helps them to know what they really want to do about their situations. [The therapist is still trying to 'sell' the therapy session to the child.]

Henry: I still don't understand. What good will it do to talk about it if they still keep on the same way ... Suppose it lasts ten or fifteen years and they keep on?

Therapist: You just wonder how long you can bear it? [This should have been the response earlier in the session.]

Henry: Yes, oh yes. [He weeps for several minutes.]

Therapist: It all looks pretty black.

Henry: [Nods] Sometimes I dream that my mother dies and that then somebody will understand me. I don't understand why I should dream that.

Therapist: You just wonder, "Will anybody ever understand me?" (Dorfman, 1976: 248–249)

We have quoted this in some detail in order to show how as the therapist begins to respond to the emotional content of what is being said, Henry is able to explore his feeling of hopelessness about being able to alter his situation. Note that the therapist avoids reassurance (often a temptation) and in the last quoted response accurately reflects Henry's depair, rather than attempting to answer the question, which would have again moved the communication away from his feeling. As Dorfman comments: "It is interesting to note that although he stated his inability to see any use in it, [Henry] made eager use of the therapist's presence." (1976: 249) (A response which in our experience is highly character-istic of adolescents.)

Another difficulty may arise because the therapist is only partially aware of what is being communicated and therefore reflects the child's feelings inaccurately as a result. In the following example, the therapist is anxious to establish the appropriate therapeutic limit, and in doing so, misses the fact that the child, by using the word "sneak", is suggesting that he recognizes that to take the toy would be wrong, but still wants it. Acknowledging this, after setting the limit, would have been more empathic, and would have helped the child to greater awareness of his feelings.

Child: [Picking up small plastic figure] Can I take just one of these, just a little one, just sneak it?

Therapist: You can't have it, because the toys are for all the children who come to the play room.

Child: There are loads more.

Therapist: But they belong here. They will be here next time for you to play with.

A dilemma which may be particularly acute for the beginner, but continues even with experience to require the exercise of fine judgements, is the extent to which the therapist should participate in the child's play. A further problem is the appropriate way in which to reflect the feelings which emerge in a child's play. These dilemmas arise both when the therapist is observing the child at play, and when the child actively seeks the therapist's participation in the activity.

We describe in chapter 4 the way in which in the early stages of Helen's therapy, the therapist made only minimal comments on her play, feeling that anything else would be too threatening. This experience is not uncommon – the therapist may also sense that the child is unready to share his play with her, or is still uncertain enough of the relationship to wish to keep his actions private. Thus for example, in the work discussed earlier with Robin, the therapist observed him taking a surreptitious suck from the baby's bottle, which he had earlier described scornfully as "just for babies", or in another example, the child played intently with some play figures kneeling with her back to the therapist. In both situations, a variety of reflections were open – the wish to drink from the bottle, uncertainty about it, the wish to keep it private, uncertainty what the therapist would think and so on. However, sensing that the child's wish for privacy was predominant, the therapist chose to respect this feeling and simply not to comment at all.

In other situations, particularly in the early stages of contact, the therapist will wish both to establish her presence, the fact that she is 'with' the child in his play, and also, if this is felt not to be too intrusive, tentatively to reflect his feelings as he plays in order to begin the process of helping him to get in touch with these and explore them. For example, in his first session, an eleven-year-old played with soldiers in a car, pushing the car along and repeating, "Let me out, let me out", later placing the soldiers in the house and fighting with them, again to the sounds of action noises. The therapist commented briefly on the feelings being expressed as he played, saying such things as "He's stuck; he really wants to get out", "They've taken over the house. It's dangerous in there with the soldiers fighting", "He really wants to escape", and so on.

Not infrequently children continue throughout their therapy to play out themes in relative isolation from the therapist. Allen, for example, describes a disturbed seven-year-old's vivid and aggressive play with houses, elephant and turtle, in which the themes of good and bad, destruction, punishment and imprisonment, were constantly played out. However, as Allen points out, the therapist's minimal responses enable the child to remain focused:

With so little sense of what any relationship could mean, Bill threw himself into a medium that made little direct use of the therapist. But he could not have done that without the steady, living, dynamic quality introduced by the person of the therapist. Without that as a background, all the material just described would again have become daydreaming, with little connection to reality. The therapist could let the phantasies be just what they were, but by his presence, his interest, his comments and the regular coming and going he could hold Bill to a reality to which he gradually felt connected. (1942: 147)

Quite commonly, however, and this usually increases as the child becomes more trustful of the relationship with the therapist, the therapist is asked to participate in the child's play, say by taking a role in a game, or joining in a board game, and so on. We discuss in chapter 4 some of the ways in which a child may use role play, but here we wish to highlight some of the factors which the therapist needs to consider in responding appropriately during such role playing.

One dilemma may arise in trying to decide how much 'body' to give to the role ascribed to the therapist by the child. Again, it may be necessary to discard the response that an adult might normally adopt in play acting with a child, where the adult may try and add to the child's enjoyment of the fantasy, or the richness of the play activity, or the child's social skills by inventing characteristics for the part, or extending the fantasy. Thus, for example, the adult, in ordinary play, being sent to get something for a dolls' tea party, might choose to return with the wrong item, confess to having forgotten what to get, or to having spilt it, and so on. In a therapeutic session, adding this kind of detail may draw the child away from the intensity of the play which is being enacted. It is important therefore, in playing out the role assigned by the child, to try and remain within the scope which the child has assigned the therapist, to check out with the child what he wishes done, and not to pre-empt this by pursuing a direction which to the adult may seem fruitful, or enjoyable. Since this may at times make the play seem more stilted than it otherwise would be, it is important to remain aware of what the child is enacting within the idiom of the play.

As we suggest in chapter 2, the therapist is often treated by the child in play in the same way that the child would treat a companion, on the same level of play as the child himself is on. It can be somewhat disconcerting to be addressed so directly, and without the reserve usually accorded to adults, unless one is aware of **why** the child is communicating in this way. The therapist is being assigned a role, and with troubled children, it is likely that this will be a subordinate one: understanding this may enable one to anticipate some of the feelings either of surprise or discomfort which may arise.

This awareness of the therapeutic purpose may also enable the therapist to avoid a slightly different pitfall, which may come from what Allen describes as "a too active and continuous participation in the actual play". (1942: 135) The difficulty here seems to arise from the fact that as the therapist becomes entirely the object of the child's projection, her own identity becomes submerged within the play, and the opportunity of reflecting the child's feelings, helping him to explore these feelings and to differentiate between his fantasy and reality, is lost.

The therapist must also be alert to the danger that, in participating in the child's play, she begins to use the play for her own therapeutic needs. In the work of one beginning therapist, for example, it was clear that the therapist in drawing a picture alongside the child, as he requested, had become absorbed in the pleasure of painting herself, and in pursuing this had become disengaged from what the child was undertaking. Or sometimes the therapist's own needs, perhaps to win in a game, or to follow the correct rules of the game may sometimes take over, and the therapeutic purpose of the shared activity is lost. One therapist, for example, attempting to play a game of draughts with a child, Katy, became more and more confused and finally irritated because the child altered the rules as the game progressed. Recognizing, in supervision, his own need for things to be correctly organized, he was able to control his feelings, and reflect his confusion to the child, making comments such as "It's hard for me to follow when I don't know where the pieces can go", "seems as if you know what's happening and I don't", until Katy finally said, as she triumphantly took the therapist's remaining piece, "I know the rules, though, so I'm all right." (This seemed a significant turning point for Katy who had experienced numerous moves in care, and when she entered therapy was confused and disturbed by her experiences. She became both more settled in her current foster home, and clearer in her wish to move to an adoptive placement, which she eventually did.)

Many of the examples we have given earlier demonstrate that in reflecting what the child is feeling, the therapist frequently addresses not merely the surface content of what is being experienced, but what she senses are the feelings underlying this. Since this is arguably a matter of interpretation, insofar as the therapist is going beyond what the child has actually said or enacted, some examination is needed of the distinctions to be made between the kind of interpretive reflection which is appropriate within non-directive therapy, and the kinds of interpretation which would occur in other forms of therapy, for example when using a psychodynamic model. It seems probable that there is a considerable overlap between the interpretive response in non-directive counselling and in other forms of psychotherapeutic intervention. What seems to be distinctive however is that in non-directive work, the therapist largely uses the idiom of the child, and responds to current feelings as the child communicates them. Unlike psychodynamic models the therapist avoids making links to events either in the child's past, or in the child's situation outside the therapy room until or unless the child makes this link himself.

Axline, in exploring the process of reflection, acknowledges the fact that much of this process involves interpretation, although she distinguishes between the two:

The child's play is symbolic of his feelings, and whenever the therapist attempts to translate symbolic behaviour into words, she is interpreting because she is saying what she **thinks** the child has expressed in actions ... even, then the therapist's response should include the **symbol** the child has used. (1987: 98)

However, although it is true that the therapist may remain entirely within the idiom of the child (talking about the baddies beating the goodies, for example, rather than personalizing the play, by attributing these feelings to those the child experiences towards his siblings) the purpose of the reflection is to assist the process of adaption and reorganization of mental schemas described in chapter 2. Although this process may remain at a low level of cognitive awareness for the child (the soldiers finding the house a dangerous place, for example) some level of conscious mental assimilation is necessary if the play is not merely to remain at the level of daydreaming described by Allen, above. Very often, the therapist by her responses will link the child's play to his mental ongoing experiences.

In reflecting his feelings the therapist tries to be aware of the nature of the child's mental defences, and only responds in a way that will help the child make the connections with other affective, motor and cognitive schemas when the child seems ready to do so.

An example may illustrate this kind of response. The following extract is from a session in which an eleven-year-old boy has just finished enacting a violent scene in the dolls house, with the play figures being wounded and thrown one by one out of the windows. The therapist was therefore aware that the theme of safety and danger was a strong current preoccupation.

> **Gerald:** That's quite dangerous on the floor. [Gerald points to a trailing flex which he moves.]
>
> **Therapist:** You think it's dangerous that the wire is there and you've moved it to make it safer.
>
> **Gerald:** Yeah – don't want people to trip over it.
>
> **Therapist:** You are looking after people by moving the wire to make sure people don't trip over it.

The therapist at this point might have helped Gerald's awareness and acknow-ledgement of his own fears by personalizing this reflection, for example, "You think it's unsafe for yourself and me". However, Gerald, after a brief diversion, returns to the theme, and directly acknowledges his own fear of the dark.

> [Gerald then moved the bean bags against the door, went over to the light switches and turned off the lights.]

Gerald: What do you think of it in here? I don't like it with the lights off. When I'm at home I call to Mum to leave the landing lights on.

Therapist: You prefer the lights to stay on all the time.

Gerald: It's frightening when the landing lights are off. [He gesticulates to the changes in the room.] What do you think of it?

Therapist: I think it makes you feel safer for it to be the way it is, and that's good.

Gerald: Yeah.

This move, from expression of a generalized, or as here, symbolic concern, to a specific personal and emotional one, is a common feature of the therapeutic process, which we discussed in more detail in chapter 4.

In another example, an eight-year-old boy living with his parents and sisters was referred by his school because of his disturbed behaviour, which vacillated in play therapy between periods of wild uncontrollable rages and withdrawn passivity. He repeatedly enacted scenes in his play where the bad play figures aggressively buried, drowned or otherwise destroyed the good figures. The therapist commented that the good figures never seemed to win, and that the bad figures were really powerful. It seemed clear from his referral that the child was dramatizing a basic conflict in his home life where he was seen as the bad child, and his siblings as good, and was punished accordingly. Had the therapist at this stage chosen to interpret this directly – you are being the bad person here and you want to get rid of your sisters – this would have gone ahead of what the child himself was aware of. When this occurs, as Axline suggests "There is the danger of thrusting something at the child before he is ready for it". (1987: 99) However, as the theme returned, the therapist then began to respond in a more directly personal way "You want the goodies shut out of the sand house" and so on; but as long as the child continued to feel it necessary to use the figures as his symbolic medium, as he did throughout the sessions, the therapist used them too.

Decisions concerning how directly to comment to a child during non-directive play therapy are often particularly acute with children's drawings and paintings. There is an extensive literature on children's paintings and their interpretation, and the reader is referred elsewhere for a fuller consideration of the subject than is possible here (see, for example, Betensky, 1973).

In responding to children's drawings, the same principles of reflection can be applied as have already been discussed, that is, the therapist should reflect the feelings being expressed in the drawing in a manner which is non-intrusive, but is sufficient to harness the drawing into current reality and, perhaps, in the early sessions to differentiate the activity of painting from the way in which it would be practised outside the therapy room. As before, the reflections are directed towards helping the child to a greater awareness of what is being expressed, while respecting the child's defence mechanisms and readiness consciously to address themes which are expressed in the paintings.

Four children's drawings (three of which are reproduced in the colour plate section) may serve to highlight specific aspects of the process, in addition to these general themes. In the first, the therapist herself is unware fully of the dynamic at work. In the second, one of her reflections is rejected at a conscious level by the child. In the third, the therapist does not reflect many of the feelings which seem to her to be expressed in the painting, since the child's demeanour suggests that this would not be congruent with what the child is consciously feeling. And in the fourth, the girl having made her painting begins consciously to explore for the first time her different feelings about her father.

In the first, Paul, aged four and a half turned to the box of felt tips towards the end of his session. He had been referred for play therapy some weeks before because of his outbursts of uncontrollable temper towards his mother. His relationship with his mother, a single parent, seemed to have deteriorated significantly since his father left home a year earlier. He was an energetic child, who spent little time with any particular toy in the play room except the clay and drawing materials.

Paul settled to drawing a train. He concentrated hard, and from the slight smile on his face and the happy air of industry was evidently enjoying what he was doing. The train was clearly drawn and brightly coloured in. The therapist reflected back to him that he liked what he had drawn, and went on to say that there were only a few minutes left before the end of their time together. Paul nodded, and took a black felt-tip pen and scribbled over his drawing of the train until it could no longer be seen.

Therapist: Black, now, on your train. Can't see the train.

Paul nodded again and continued quickly and thoughtfully to cover the train completely. This did not seem to be done in anger, or with anything but careful thought. The therapist felt perplexed. Paul put the black pen down, and looked pleased with the result.

Therapist: Now your train's gone and you're happy.

Paul liked his mother to bring him to his play therapy sessions and collect him. She came into the room at the end of the hour. She noticed his drawing and in the child's presence expressed her concern to the therapist: "Oh dear, what does all that black mean? Do you think he's depressed, do you think he's getting worse?"

Paul glanced up at the therapist with twinkling eyes. The therapist felt then that she had understood: Paul had finally managed to achieve some privacy in his life, away from his mother who was rather intrusive. He left the session with an amused and triumphant smile.

This illustrates the potential pitfalls in interpreting the child's activity: although the therapist follows the child's lead it may not always result in her full understanding of the play. Nonetheless, in this example, because of the therapist's respect for the child's privacy he seemed to achieve what was necessary for him, even while it was only incompletely understood by the therapist.

Edward, aged twelve, had been seeing the play therapist for many months. He and other members of his family had been sexually abused by his stepfather, who had received a prison sentence. There had been press coverage of the case, and as a result of the abuse becoming general knowledge he was frequently bullied by his peer group at the village school he attended.

He often came to the therapy session with apparently little idea of what use he would make of the materials on offer, and sometimes sat and thought about what he might do for half the session. During this session, having scanned the content of the room and reassured himself that everything was in its place, he began to draw. His drawing was rather scribbly, at times chaotic, which seemed to reflect his feelings and his family life. Despite the fact that his drawing was ostensibly of a fishing trip on a sunny day, it had a sense of grimness about it (Plate 4).

> **Therapist:** Two people in the boat, looking very serious, sort of grim.
>
> **Edward:** They're fishing ... there's a good place to go fishing nearby here. I go a lot, at night, after school.

As he drew, he talked of the previous evening's fishing. Three boys had crept up on him as he fished from the bank. They had pushed him into the river and refused to let him climb out. He had been in the water for an hour before an adult passing by had intervened. His hands shook as he drew and he looked near to tears. He then drew a building with a tower and rudimentary battlements.

> **Therapist:** And a big building, down by the river.
>
> **Edward:** That's my school – it isn't really so near to the river, but it's quite near.
>
> **Therapist:** Drawing of your school, and it's almost like a church – like a big church by the river.
>
> **Edward:** [looked puzzled] Well, it's my school.

The therapist wondered whether to reflect further to the child concerning the school, but as he had not picked up on her comment about the similarity to a church decided not to. She was aware that religion held a very central place in his life, and that the values of forgiveness and acceptance were strongly maintained by his mother. This created obvious conflicts for him. His stepfather had abused him, which had in part provoked the continual bullying at school, isolating him even though the abuse had ended. Despite this, he was admonished to forgive and accept. The fusion of the two images of school and church in the drawing suggest that perhaps at some level this conflict was being addressed. Even though he consciously rejected the therapist's reflection, it seems possible that the creation of the drawing, coupled with the therapist's comment, enabled him to begin to explore these conflicts, since in subsequent sessions they emerged repeatedly and he was able to explore this theme more directly.

Hilary, age nine, found it difficult to make any decision in the play therapy session, feeling safer if the therapist made the choice about what she should do.

> **Hilary:** What shall I do today?
>
> **Therapist:** Just wondering.
>
> **Hilary:** You say.
>
> **Therapist:** You'd rather I tell you.
> [Hilary stopped for a moment. Then]
>
> **Hilary:** Will you draw a bear for me?

She often asked the therapist to draw for her because her own drawings were "no good", but on this occasion, as the therapist drew, there was a change.

> **Hilary:** That bear looks like a human.
>
> **Therapist:** Not really the way you wanted it.

Helen then took over the drawing herself. She carefully drew and painstakingly coloured her bear in, giving it black hair and blue eyes. It looked very human (Plate 5).

> **Hilary:** Bears can be nice sometimes, sometimes they can be frightening.
>
> **Therapist:** Bears not always the same, they can change.
>
> **Hilary:** The bear is my dad.
>
> **Therapist:** Dad can be different as well.
>
> **Hilary:** Dad is horrible. [Wistfully] Sometimes I would like to see him.

For the first time, she seemed able to put her conflicting feelings about her father beside one another, which until this moment she had been unable to do. Previously her feelings about her father had been idealized, saying that if he would only come back to live with the family, things would be better. She went on to draw flowers beside the bear, saying that she wanted to make it look nice. The therapist reflected that she "wanted to make the bear look nice and feel nicer". Hilary still retained a strong sense of responsibility for the abuse and the break-up of the family. Decorating the drawing with flowers communicated vividly to the therapist that she still felt that she was the one who should make things better, but to have reflected this would have been to go beyond what Hilary, at this point, was able herself to acknowledge.

Becky, aged seven, seemed from her appearance and behaviour to be a much younger child. Initially, and for many sessions subsequently, she had remained standing, still and silent, unable to play with any of the materials present. The therapist made few reflections, as Becky indicated by covering her ears, that she did not want her to talk much; she would turn her back or put her arm around her drawing, as if to guard against intrusion. Some way into therapy, she began to draw the picture illustrated in Plate 6. (Note that the painting suggests the work of a much younger child.) She drew it with great urgency, energy and concentration in a manner which was in stark contrast to her lack of energy and activity earlier. On this occasion, too, she seemed happy for the therapist to see her picture.

> **Therapist:** Lots of colours. Red, green, yellow.
> [Becky nodded.]
>
> **Becky:** That's me. [She indicated the pink smiling figure in the drawing.]
>
> **Therapist:** You're in your picture . . . smiling.

Becky continued to draw quickly and intently. She indicated that the purple-faced, black figure was her father.

> **Therapist:** Dad, smiling too. Long, thin dad, black inside.

The therapist felt concerned, looking at the drawing of dad, that it might have another meaning, as it was an obviously phallic shape and there had already been worries and some signs that Becky had been sexually abused. However, there was no indication from the child's manner, or in her voice, that she was worried, or frightened about "dad". The therapist did not share these concerns with the child: they arose from her adult interpretation of the painting, which seemed to be supported by her knowledge of the child's history. Becky, however, showed no sign of conscious recognition of negative feelings, and to have gone further with the reflection would have been to risk confusing her, confronting her defences, and being overly suggestive.

Finally, in this section, we should emphasize again the importance attached to the therapist's alertness to her own patterns of responses to the child in therapy. At a straightforward level, it is sensible to be aware of one's own predilections and reservations: for example, if the physical sensation of clay is personally unpleasant, it is better not to include this in the play equipment rather than to struggle to overcome feelings of distaste at handling it, which will undoubtedly impede the ability to respond accurately to the child's play. Many adults are disturbed by a great deal of mess and disorder: although if the need for orderliness is very considerable, play therapy may not be an appropriate method to adopt, it is proper to take some steps to reduce the possibility of mess (we discuss the therapeutic setting of limits in the following section). We have already discussed the need to unlearn for the purposes of therapy some of the responses which are entirely appropriate to adult–child exchanges in a different context (the protecting, stimulating, educating responses). Attitudes concerning permissiveness, discipline or views that children should be self-stimulating (that is, that they 'should' be able to play on their own), a tendency towards competitiveness or a need to win may be more difficult responses to anticipate until they emerge within the therapeutic encounter, and a willingness to address these in supervision is essential.

Many therapists have at times to struggle with the intrusiveness of other thoughts during the play session; this may occur, for example, in situations where the therapist is experiencing personal stress, or after a particularly difficult encounter at work. It may be appropriate to acknowledge that one is somewhat abstracted, since it is likely that the child will sense this anyway. However, it seems best not to be over specific in this: for example, an explanation to a child about a missed appointment, occasioned by the sudden acute illness of the therapist's mother, brought a hostile "Well *I* managed to get here." The therapist in retrospect felt that although she had considered that knowing the circumstances behind the cancellation would make it more acceptable, the child did not want to think of her except in relation to him, and was burdened by the additional information.

Intrusive sexual thoughts, or sexual responses, to the child's sexualized behaviour in therapy, are in our experience often disturbing and difficult to deal with and we discuss these in more detail in chapter six. Here we should note that we do not consider that it is ever appropriate to share these with the child, whether their source is personal material triggered by the child's behaviour, or a direct response to it unless in the exceptional circumstance cited above.

Finally, many therapists from time to time have to struggle to overcome feelings of boredom and lack of interest in what the child is doing. This may be a reflection of something the child is experiencing, since children not uncommonly go through periods, usually brief, of not wanting to do anything, feeling dissatisfied with what they have been doing, and so on. It is important here for the therapist to use her feelings congruently with the child. Sometimes this lack of interest may in fact be an indication that the therapy is coming to a natural end; more frequently, it is an emotion which can disguise something else – anger or frustration, for example, that are as yet too threatening to acknowledge; or the therapist may not have helped the child sufficiently to focus on what is troubling him. Sometimes, however, it is a more personal feeling on the part of the therapist, and may have its source in a lack of faith in the approach itself. Because much of what the child does is at a nonverbal and symbolic level, it may take time before it is possible to discern much pattern or meaning in the play, and for observable change to occur. Good supervision, and a willingness to scrutinize the protocols of the therapy sessions, may help to overcome this difficulty.

SECTION TWO

ESTABLISHING LIMITS

Determining the appropriate level of permissiveness to be established within the therapeutic session can be problematic, and as we suggest in chapter 3 it is important to consider as far as one can before therapy begins which limits will need to be imposed and how they are to be introduced. Although some restrictions exist in all therapies the establishment of limits is particularly an issue in non-directive therapy because it is conducted in a context which is generally more permissive than in the world outside the play room, and is one in which children are encouraged to express feelings freely, and in ways which might in a different context be unacceptable. There may seem to be in inherent tension in an approach which says on the one hand, express and explore your feelings, and on the other, beyond this point in your behaviour you may not go. This section explores this paradox; the practical and therapeutic reasons for imposing limits; the way in which limits in therapy may differ from those in a non-therapeutic context; and the issues arising from the introduction of those limits.

The guiding principles for the use of limits in non-directive therapy are that they both should reflect the practical reality of the constraints imposed by the physical context in which the therapy is conducted, and should also address the therapeutic needs of the child. In relation to the latter, the skill needed is to establish a level of permissiveness which is sufficient to allow the child to express and explore feelings freely, and at the same time to set boundaries to the child's behaviour which will both offer a sense of security and the potential for certain therapeutic experiences.

Non-directive therapists consistently stress the need for limits, although they acknowledge that therapists will vary in the level of restrictions which they impose. Axline, for example, in a chapter which offers much useful advice and to which the reader is referred, argues that at a pragmatic level limits need to be established:

Also, commonsense limitations which are necessary for the protection of the child should be included. There seems to be little or no therapeutic value in spending a play period with the child hanging out of a high window or engaging in any activity that is dangerous to him. If he is to come out of the therapy room with a feeling of security and respect for the therapist, he must be treated in such a manner, while in the room with the therapist, that these feelings are built up. (1987: 128)

Quite apart from the dubious benefits to the child in not doing so, it seems clear that behaviour needs to be restricted which has damaging practical consequences, for example, which involves breaking toys, fixtures and fittings, which have to be replaced, removing items of equipment which are then not available for other children.

Given that the limits imposed must partly reflect practical circumstances, it is inevitable that the level of permissive behaviour will vary according to the particular demands of the setting. It is likely too that the personal expectations, style and preferences of the therapist will have some impact on limits within which the therapy is conducted, given different levels of tolerance of mess, noise and so on. (Although as we suggest elsewhere, a need for orderliness beyond a certain level might indicate an unsuitability for this method of working with children.)

The limits which arise from practical circumstances commonly concern such things as breaking toys, equipment or furniture, taking toys home, painting on the walls, leaving the play room (because at a practical level it may interrupt others working in the building), playing with the tape recorder, or the therapist's spectacles, handbag etc., and behaviour which may endanger or harm the child, or hurt the therapist. However, there are likely to be a myriad of activities which come into a rather grey area, where the therapist may feel uncertain about whether the behaviour needs to be checked: does it matter, for example, if a child proceeds to paint the dolls house, easel, or the wooden legs of a chair, puts the soft toys in the tub of water so they will be wet for the next session with a different child, dollops finger paints on the floor covering, and so on? It is difficult to anticipate all these things in advance, and often the therapist has to take a quick decision, balancing the needs of the individual child with the needs and expectations and possible disapproval of others who will use the room. The therapist's uncertainty over limits is likely both to communicate itself unhelpfully to the child, and also to obstruct the therapist's focus on the child's therapeutic needs. For this reason, it is very much easier, if at all possible, to conduct the sessions in a room with which one is familiar, and where the constraints are known and can be anticipated. It goes without saying that it is also much easier to use a purpose built playroom, where there is less likelihood of damaging the setting, and less anxiety about what other people will think.

Although this may not always be the case (since unfortunately some settings may require constraints which one feels unhelpfully restrict the child), many limits will have a dual purpose, in being imposed for both practical and therapeutic reasons. The restriction on self-harm for example, will serve therapeutically to convey the therapist's concern for the child's safety and well being; the limits of time, which may arise from practical constraints on what the therapist is able to offer, lends a structure and sense of safety to the therapeutic situation for a child and hence reduces his feelings of anxiety engendered by the experience. The regularity of the time at which the session is held, and the consistency of the setting also provides a safe boundary in which the child's feelings are contained, and may help the child to experience the therapist as a reliable and consistent figure.

This notion that in order to be able to explore feelings safely the individual needs to feel securely held, and that this sense of security is conveyed in concrete terms by certain boundaries on the therapeutic encounter is widely accepted in the literature (eg Moustakas, 1953; Dorfman, 1976; see also Reisman, 1973, for the therapeutic relevance of limits in other psycho-therapeutic approaches). Reisman, for example, suggests that they are helpful "for both child and therapist, by affording some assurance that certain things cannot be done". (1973: 45) They also provide a means of anchoring the therapy in the world of reality, at moments when the individual may be fearful of being overwhelmed by frightening feelings, of going crazy, and losing touch with reality.

However, limits used in play therapy have a therapeutic function over and above the establishment for a child of a sense of safety and reality which appears to have received little acknowledgement in the literature: namely, that limits provide one means whereby the child gains mastery over his feelings.

How may this be so? There are a number of facets, or stages, involved in the process, which allow the child to assimilate the experience into existing schemas, in the ways outlined in chapter 2. First, in being denied something, the child experiences in concrete terms, around the specific event, feelings of wanting and not having, of which he is consciously aware. (The child knows, for example, that he wants to break the dolls house or to keep the glove puppet for himself.) Second, the therapist recognizes and accepts the child's feelings about being denied the desired object or activity, and, sometimes, the child's wish to break the rule. ("You really want badly to take the puppet home, but you can't.") Third, by communicating this and importantly communicating acceptance of this desire, the therapist helps to make the feelings conscious, so that the child can allow the feeling about this concrete event to merge into other feelings which he has had, or may still have, about related experiences. And fourth, in re-enacting these conscious feelings in play, the child is able to put the experiences and associated feelings into a wider context.

This sequence may occur repeatedly within the child's behaviour in therapy. Ben, for example, at intervals over a period of weeks, asked to be given more soldiers, more drink, more time in the play room (taxing the therapist considerably, incidentally, who found it difficult not to accede to his requests).

When his feelings were acknowledged, but at the same time he was told he could not have more, he proceeded in a variety of ways to play out his feelings of anger and sense of deprivation: burying figures in the sand, drowning them, shutting them up in the cupboard and so on. After some time, he began to feed the toy animals with the baby bottle; finally, he began to feed himself, saying as he did so, "I'm feeding myself; it's all for me, now." This feeling that he needed more than he had was reflected in his everyday behaviour and he began to discuss being adopted with his social worker and foster parents, an issue he adamantly refused to countenance previously.

Not all children of course use limits therapeutically in this way in their play. Our practice experience suggests that limit setting is most likely to enable the child to address other related feelings when the child is one who has expressed his unhappiness through acting-out forms of behaviour, probably linked to a deep seated sense of deprivation: Ben's behaviour, for example, was reported by school and foster parents to be often wild and uncontrollable (although he did not, in fact, behave in this way in therapy, adopting instead other testing behaviour which was less physically demanding). An over punitive and at the same time withholding regime with his natural parents perhaps made it more predictable that this would be an area which he needed to explore emotionally.

The way in which limits are established is important. We have already suggested, in chapter 3, that at the outset it is unnecessary and may even be inappropriate to say more about these beyond giving an indication of the duration of the session and the time, day and number of sessions which the child is offered. When the need arises, it is important to set the limit first, so that the child understands this clearly; then to acknowledge and reflect that the child wants what he cannot have (or must not do), if this is an accurate reflection of what the child is feeling.

> **Tom:** Can I take one of these finger puppets home?
>
> **Therapist:** No, the things are for you to play with here, not take home. It's really hard for you when I say no, and you want it badly.
> Tom here plays out aggression and anger with the toy soldiers and the sand, and then tries to extend the limits again:
>
> **Tom:** Can I stay an hour and a quarter?
>
> **Therapist:** No, just the hour. It is hard for you when I say only an hour, because you want to stay longer. Difficult for you, just like the biscuits [of which he has also earlier asked for more] when I say no more, when you want more. [The therapist appropriately links the child's concrete experiences within the session, of not having enough. Tom then enacts a further complex aggressive sequence of play.]

Note that the therapist's acknowledgement of the feeling, and the communication that this is understood and accepted by her, is an important part of the sequence. As we suggested in the previous section it is also important to keep the reflection short, or it becomes less effective, and the highly emotive content is lessened. The therapist must also have an internal commitment to establishing the limit, since ambivalence is quickly picked up by the child, as we illustrated in the over complex response to the child's request to take a toy from the playroom, quoted in the last section.

These themes are not necessarily communicated verbally: particularly with very young children, the communication may remain largely at a non-verbal level, with the therapist gently taking whatever action is appropriate to demonstrate to the child what the rule is.

Children may need clarification as to what they are allowed to do in the playroom, since they are understandably trying to make sense of what is, after all, an unfamiliar experience. As we suggest in chapter 4, it is helpful to acknowledge this difference, and to explain that it is possible to do some things in the playroom which are not permitted outside, since this clarifies for the child that things are different, and avoids giving apparent support to behaviour which may be forbidden elsewhere. In response, for example, to a hesitant look of enquiry from the child, the therapist might say "You're wondering if it's all right to do that. It is OK. You can do some things in here which you can't do outside."

Since concern is sometimes expressed that this level of permissiveness will lead to misbehaviour on the part of the child outside therapy, it is worth noting that with therapeutic help children appear very quickly to recognize and accept the differences between the two contexts, and do not tend to carry out behaviour (tipping sand on to the floor, for example) into a different setting. (As we suggest in chapter 3, the child's behaviour outside therapy may in fact initially pose more of a management problem. For example, bedwetting, nightmares, demanding behaviour may become more pronounced, but the reason for this seems to lie in the surfacing of hitherto unacknowledged feelings, rather than a blurring of rules between the playroom and his other environments.)

A child may do something that he suspects may be wrong, or which the therapist will be annoyed by. Equally, he may go ahead and break a rule of which he has just been reminded, or one which he knows about but has probably forgotten. In each of these different circumstances, it is important to reflect what the child is feeling, as well as clarifying what is permissible. Where the child does seem intent on doing something which he knows he should not, the therapist does need, ultimately, to establish control, physically restraining the child if necessary, and stating that the session will end and bringing it to a close if the child persists. As Axline's comment quoted at the beginning of the section suggests, there is little therapeutic gain for the child if the therapist loses control of the session in this way.

It is, ultimately, the therapist's responsibility to ensure that the child does not break a particular rule, especially since, as we have suggested, it is important for him to have a sense of being securely held in therapy. Mistakes do sometimes occur, either because the therapist has failed to anticipate something quickly enough, or if, for example, the child accidentally breaks something. In these circumstances, it may be sometimes appropriate for the therapist to acknowledge to the child her feeling of responsibility for what has occurred.

Another issue arises in relation to the child who tries to extend the limits, but does so within the metaphor of his play: for example, in a scene in which the child was enacting a complex battle with the therapist as opponent, he began firing clay pellets directly at her; in another, where an eight-year-old boy had been role playing scenes between his mother and a succession of boyfriends, with the therapist taking the part of the mother, the boy started to bind her to her chair (whether mimicking what he observed, or symbolically representing what he was feeling, was obscure). In both examples, the play was clearly interrupted by the therapists' setting the limit. They were therefore concerned lest the therapeutic value of the play would be lost. It nonetheless seemed vital to retain the appropriate limit on the child's freedom, not least, in the latter example, because the potential loss of control by the therapist would have ultimately been unhelpful to the child. (A distinction, however, should be made between this, where the therapist risks losing physical control, and a role play in which the therapist may enact a role of being helpless.)

We conclude with an observation by Axline which summarizes many of the therapeutic reasons for using limits within the therapy sessions:

It seems that limitations used with intelligence and consistency serve to anchor the therapy session to the world of reality and to safeguard the therapy from possible misconceptions, confusion, guilt feelings, and insecurity. It is the principle that serves as a device by which the child's participation, co-operation, and responsibility can be measured. It is the principle that calls forth all the tact, consistency, honesty, and strength of the therapist. (1987: 134)

In this section, we have considered both the therapeutic and practical reasons for imposing limits in the therapeutic session, and discussed some of the practice skills involved in this. In the following section, we consider another dilemma which may arise in therapeutic work when a child makes a disclosure of abuse.

| S E C T I O N   T H R E E |

ISSUES CONCERNING DISCLOSURE AND VALIDATION

A dilemma may arise for the therapist conducting non-directive play therapy when the child discloses that he is being abused, or makes a further and fuller disclosure during therapy. As was pointed out in evidence in Cleveland "after the discovery of abuse, at least in outline form, then it is quite possible that there will be further disclosure within the context of therapeutic involvement with the child and the family ..." (Butler-Sloss, 1988: 208) Although more attention has been paid to the problem of validating information in cases of child sexual abuse, it is not uncommon for the child to reveal evidence of other forms of abuse which suggest the need for investigation and possible protective action; the difficulties posed for the therapist are similar. These concern the need to preserve the child's trust in the therapeutic relationship while cutting across its private nature; the need to be clear in one's own mind about the distinction between validation and work with a therapeutic purpose; and the need to consider who should conduct the validation interview. Related to these concerns are those about whether it is appropriate to maintain the non-directive approach in other contacts with the child, which we discuss at the end of the section.

On occasion, the child's first experience of the therapist may be in the context of a validation interview. If the child experiences the interview as in some way enabling and supportive, then the process of engagement with the child and the beginning of trust may have occurred. This may quite appropriately lead into non-directive therapy in order to explore, if the child wishes, the feelings around some of the experiences the child has been sharing.

It is however important, as we suggest in our discussion of the use of play for diagnostic purposes, to recognize the different nature of validation and therapeutic work (whatever model is adopted in the latter). It is true that a validation interview, sensitively conducted, may provide some relief from the burden of the abuse, and the acknowledgement of the child's feelings about it may be a source of emotional strength. There are other similarities between the two: both the validation interview and any subsequent therapeutic intervention must have a clear professional remit and purpose, be set within time boundaries, and recognize the limits of confidentiality.

Nonetheless a validation interview contrasts with a therapeutic session in being a purposeful, information gathering exercise which strives to produce an evidentially sound exchange which can be reported to the court in either civil or criminal proceedings. The questions are open rather than leading, but have a definite structure to them. The investigators' main task is to ascertain what, if anything, has happened, how, with whom, where, whether any witnesses were present who might corroborate the child's account, and whether there is a possibility of medical evidence. The interview is organized around the inter-viewers' agenda rather than the child's, for even when children have made a purposeful, intentional, disclosure, they are rarely eager to discuss the various incidents in the detail the interviewer requires. Guidelines issued following **Cleveland** suggest that two validation interviews are acceptable (more possibly becoming harmful to the child, and being of little value evidentially). The interviews should be of no more than forty-five minutes to one hour fifteen minutes, depending on the age of the child. The anatomically complete dolls, once regarded so confidently, are now viewed as evidentially unsound unless used much later in the interviewing process. Even then they should only be used after the child has made a clear disclosure, in order to enable the child to act out with the dolls in a concrete way what he may be struggling to find words to express. Certainly Yuille, whose step-wise approach to interviewing has found an advocate in the Pigot Report, considers any toys, drawing materials, books etc. as unhelpful in terms of gathering evidentially uncontaminated information from the child, and suggests that they should only be resorted to when verbal communication alone has failed (Report of the Advisory Group on Video Evidence, 1989).

There are still likely to be two investigating officers present at a validation interview, although research suggests that a single interviewer may be more effective. The issue of the gender of the investigating officer has recently been acknowledged and where possible the child is given a choice of male or female interviewer. Finally, the session is increasingly likely to be video-taped, normally without obtaining the child's permission.

There are clear differences in purpose and process between this and the therapeutic intervention, particularly in the context of this book. The content of each session in non-directive play therapy is unstructured, facilitated by one adult and not two, and the building of a relationship between child and therapist, which is fundamental to the therapeutic process, is at the child's and not the therapist's pace. The number of sessions offered to the child in therapy is largely determined by the child's needs, rather than concern about producing evidentially sound interviews. A non-directive play session, properly conducted, should, as we discuss later in this chapter, produce evidentially valid information, but can never be directed towards filling in gaps in the information held.

We highlight these distinctions in order to underline the very real dilemmas posed for the therapist when abuse is revealed during the course of therapeutic work, since it will be clear that very different techniques and purposes are involved in the two activities. These dilemmas are threefold, concerning confidentiality, the extent to which a (partial) disclosure is pursued, and who should undertake the disclosure work. As Glaser and Frosh succinctly point out:

Questions arise both in relation to confidentiality, which is necessary for the psychotherapeutic relationship to be maintained, and in relation to technique, which may well have been reflective and interpretive, rather than investigative. Pursuing the abuse might jeopardise the therapy, yet there is a need to protect the child. If it is believed that abuse is continuing, it is unlikely that disclosure by itself will lead to cessation of the abuse. (1988: 76)

It is important, as we suggested in chapter 3, to discuss at the beginning of the sessions the possibility that information may need to be shared with others if issues of protecting the child or other children arise. However, it will be readily understood that this does not necessarily remove the difficulty from the child's point of view: the extent to which the child is able to 'hear' such a statement before it becomes meaningful as a live issue, must be variable, and although the child's feelings of having his trust betrayed are undoubtedly ameliorated by the therapist's referring back to her earlier statement, they may not wholly be dispelled.

Moreover, the child is frequently resistant to the idea that the information disclosed needs to be taken further. Although on occasion the child does divulge abuse in order that some action be taken over it, or may come later to accept this, this is rarely the initial impulse for disclosure. The child, speaking for the first time, may only be aware of the wish to unburden himself of a heavy secret, or may, as Glaser and Frosh suggest, be "testing the safety of an outsider's response". The statement may be made from an overwhelming wish at that moment for the abuse to stop, or much more frequently, in a younger child, a statement may be made to relieve the child of some of the anxiety/ discomfort resulting from the abuse, and without a full understanding of the impact and implications such a statement may have on the therapist. (This of course is similar to other situations considered earlier, where the adult has much fuller knowledge of the implications of the child's actions or statements than the child.)

Rachel, age fifteen, had been sexually abused for some years by her father before finally revealing another assault. The therapist noted:

During an early session with Rachel she said she was going to talk to me about something she had not told anyone before. She told me that she had been raped, in her foster placement, by a visitor to the home. Because of the devastating experience of giving evidence at her father's trial, she had decided not to tell anyone about the sexual assault, and had instead run away from the foster home. I said at this point that I might not be able to keep the information she wanted to share with me just to myself.

She looked troubled and irritated with me. I reflected these feelings: "You're wondering why our time together will be different, why I can't just keep everything to myself?"

Rachel sighed heavily: "All I want is to have someone to talk to who won't go telling everyone else about my life."

The information she went on to share related to an incident that had happened some years before. She did not name the boy, and was adamant that she did not wish to make any sort of complaint, without which the police would in any case be unable to pursue an investigation.

In this example, the therapist's (and the child's) position was relatively straightforward, in that the abuse was no longer current and Rachel was old enough to recognize, when the therapist alerted her to them, the implications of what she was saying, and be clear about what she wanted to do. Even here, however, a professional judgement had to be made about whether or not to seek more information, in particular because of the potential risk to other children. This judgement involved the weighing up of Rachel's therapeutic needs against the uncertainties of invoking an investigative procedure.

In other circumstances, the form of the child's disclosure may leave the therapist with no alternative but to share the information with colleagues. We have two reasons for saying this: first, although therapists in non-statutory settings may have greater freedom over the decision, in many instances, particularly for social workers in statutory settings, their agency's remit may require that the disclosure is reported. Second, if the abuse is on-going, the therapeutic work on its own will not be sufficient to help the child, or to counteract the impact of the abusive relationship(s) in which the child is involved. (See discussion of the timing of therapy in chapter 3.)

The timing of such action on the part of the therapist must again be a matter for professional judgement. In some circumstances, the release of feelings engendered by the disclosure during therapy may in the therapist's view put the child at some immediate risk, either of physical harm, or of serious and frightening pressure from the abuser to retract the statement. In such cases, the therapist may decide that immediate action is required (and indeed sometimes the child himself asks to come into care, or to be removed from the abusive situation).

In other circumstances, and particularly where the child is resistant to the therapist divulging the disclosure, the therapist may decide to spend time exploring the child's feelings concerning the abuse, and helping the child prepare for the investigation. (But see next section for the importance of not 'contaminating' the child's evidence.) It is clearly important, if such a course of action is pursued, that the therapist is purposive, and does not allow the child to lose sight of the eventual need for the disclosure to be reported elsewhere. It may also be strategically wise for the statutory therapist to inform her line manager of the situation, while preserving the child's confidence. In the long run, it is likely that any child protection process will be more effective if the child can be empowered in this way, since he will be less likely to retract or to be made to feel helpless during the process.

A six-year-old boy, Jamie, disclosed during play therapy that a black eye of some weeks ago had been caused by a punch from his stepfather. Previous questioning by a teacher and social worker and a medical examination had not elicited this information, and the boy went on to reveal a succession of harsh punishments for misbehaviour inflicted on him by his parents. He was frightened and very reluctant to have the information divulged. The therapist, while making it clear that she would need to do so soon, spent the next session exploring this with him, balancing what she felt was important for him in terms of preparation against the possible risks that could accrue from this delay.

When a child makes a partial disclosure, or the therapist remains unclear about what has been said, some hesitation may be felt about whether or not to move from a non-directive stance in order to clarify what is being communicated. The difficulty may arise because the therapist experiences a tension between a need to continue to help the child explore what he is saying or doing, and the need to establish, for child protection purposes, what has happened. Usually, in our experience, these two purposes are not, in fact, incompatible: for example, if a child draws a picture of a figure in a posture suggestive of abuse (as in Plate 6) clarifying who the adult figure in the picture represents may be done in a way which is consistent with a non-directive approach, in that it is perfectly appropriate for the therapist to wish to make sense of what is being portrayed in order the better to understand it and the feelings surrounding it.

There may however come a point where the two purposes clearly diverge, and it is at this stage of the process that the therapist is faced with the dilemma of what to do. It is difficult to make a hard and fast rule about this, and it is important for the therapist to be guided by her professional judgement of what, in the particular situation, seems to be in the child's best interests.

Finally, and perhaps most frequently of all in therapy, no 'disclosure' as such is involved, but the child's play, drawings, or behaviour in the session is strongly suggestive of the fact that he is, or has been, in an abusive or damaging situation. Such a conclusion on the part of the therapist can only, in these situations, be a matter of inference, and may vary from a cumulative impression, built up over a number of sessions, that the child is experiencing emotional abuse within his family setting, to an assessment drawn from one or more specific episodes within therapy. In these circumstances, it is unlikely that the therapist will need to depart from a non-directive stance within the therapeutic exchange. However, the sharing of this professional opinion, based on what has been inferred in the session, does involve some breaching of confidentiality, and should certainly be discussed with the child. The ways in which children respond to this vary enormously. Often with a small child, little needs to be said, and although on the whole we would say something briefly, one needs to be sure that this is prompted by an assessment of what is in the child's interests, and not by a personal wish for honesty at all costs. Older children may want to know in greater detail what is going to be said, and although often, and perhaps usually, the information can be shared with their acceptance and indeed positive support, sadly this is not always the case. Deciding on a course of action because one feels it is in the child's long-term interests to do so, in the knowledge that this may adversely affect the therapeutic relationship, is not easy: we can only acknowledge the painfulness of the dilemma first to ourselves and then use these feelings congruently by sharing them with the child.

CONDUCTING THE VALIDATION INTERVIEW

Where the child in therapy discloses information which does require further investigation, the question of whether or not the therapist should herself participate in the validation process requires careful consideration. One may argue that the child in sharing the information has placed his trust in the therapist and that the relationship already established will facilitate the investigative process. Sadly, too, such interviews are not always conducted in a properly child-centred manner, as events in Rochdale and the Orkneys have shown, and in such situations the therapist's involvement may act as an insurance against intrusive questioning. Nonetheless, the involvement by the therapist is likely to have a profound effect on the subsequent relationship with the child. Attempting to move back again into a therapeutic role having acted as investigator is likely to create further confusion for the child, and may seriously damage any trust established (see Jones and Krugman, 1986).

This is particularly the case when the validation interview has not been, as perhaps the child hoped it would be, a relief and in itself therapeutic. Children and adults alike are often under the misconception that a validation interview, that is, sharing the fact of the abusive experience, is of itself helpful. Not surprisingly, we would like to hold on to this notion, as it is more comforting for adults, but the discovery for the child that this is not so in his own case, can in itself cause more anger and pain, anger which may be directed at the therapist for having allowed it to happen.

> **Jan:** All these years I've thought it would be a relief in the end to say. These programmes on TV talk about you feeling better when you've told. Everyone's telling me now I'll feel better because I've said, and I don't, I feel worse. There's no relief, it feels worse. The nightmares have come back. It's worse than before.

> **Therapist:** Feeling angry and let down. You thought it was going to get better, everyone told you it would get better and it's worse.

> **Jan:** And I don't feel the same here any more. It's spoilt.

> **Therapist:** Wishing that this could have remained the same. But it hasn't.

Other sources have stressed the danger of confusing the two processes. In his evidence to the Cleveland Inquiry, for example, Jones states:

An attempt to encourage disclosure while providing therapeutic treatment is fraught with difficulty ... I am opposed to treatment and 'disclosure' proceeding in parallel. (Butler-Sloss, 1988: 208)

Because of the potential risk of confusion for the child, the difficulties for the therapist and for the child protection process itself, our tentative conclusion is that it is more appropriate for the validation interview to be conducted by someone other than the therapist.

WHERE SHOULD THE NON-DIRECTIVE APPROACH BEGIN AND END?

This section has focused on the need which the therapist may sometimes have to move from a non-directive stance, and the dilemmas that this may pose. Problems may also arise for therapists who have contact with the child outside the therapeutic session concerning whether or not to maintain an exclusively non-directive approach.

Children do in fact seem to accept readily enough that the time spent together in counselling will be of a different nature to the time spent outside the sessions. However, if the therapist is the person who is transporting the child to and from the therapy session, it does seem to make sense, particularly to the child, to use a non-directive approach throughout.

Sometimes substantive issues may be addressed during the journey before the therapy session actually begins, and then may be left by the child, perhaps completely, or at least until the end of the session.

David, for example, age three, began to talk to the therapist as he travelled home with his mother beside him, of an abusive experience which he had had involving her some two years before. She was clearly shocked and had no idea that he had memories of this happening. She laughed nervously and tried to dismiss what he was saying, but the clear piping voice continued, accurately recounting his mother's attempt to suffocate him, an event recorded in the agency file at the time, but never explored with the child until now.

> **Therapist:** You remember what happened then. Mum's saying you've got it wrong.

> **David:** Well she did. She did try to.

Having been explored for a few minutes during the journey this was never referred to again by the child, although the mother continued with her denial of the incident long after the journey was over. In this instance, there seemed little to be gained by seeking further to clarify what the child had recounted. Circumstantial evidence indicated that the incident had occurred some time before. No action had been taken then, the child was in the therapist's view properly protected now, and even had criminal proceedings been contemplated, as in different circumstances they might have been, the child's statement would not have been admissible in evidence.

However, on occasion the child may disclose on the journey to his session information which is, for the kinds of reasons discussed above, important to clarify. In these circumstances, the therapist should do this, even if it means diverging from the non-directive approach customarily adopted.

We have in this section considered the dilemmas which may arise for the therapist where the possible need for protective action occurs during the period of therapeutic work. We consider in the final section the related issue of presenting therapeutic work in a court setting.

PRESENTING THERAPEUTIC WORK IN A COURT SETTING

Since many of the children referred for therapeutic help are likely to be the subject of statutory intervention, the therapist may at some point be required to present an account to the court of the therapeutic work undertaken. We write at a time (July 1991) when recent events in Rochdale and Orkney have highlighted some of the pitfalls involved for professionals in giving evidence in court concerning their direct work with children. Although criticism has largely been directed at those giving evidence arising from investigations rather than therapy, some discussion is appropriate of the most helpful way to present therapeutic work in a context which is, at best, unclear about its nature and, at worst, critical of it. We discuss some of these issues by reference to a specific hypothetical report.

Non-directive work is particularly suited to the kind of climate within which child-care practitioners are now working, since although, as we make clear in chapter 1, it makes no claim to be a method of working which is totally neutral or free from suggestion, it is non-interpretive, and the therapist follows the child's lead rather than directing the child's play. She does not ask information-seeking questions, or influence the activity by interpretations (which may be seen as suggestive). When the child's play, activity or verbal communication is reported, therefore, it is possible to identify these as spontaneous rather than as the result of the therapist's desire that the child should play or talk about a specific topic.

This is not, of course, to say that the therapist makes no interpretive comment in her report or in her statements to the court: on the contrary. Although it will be possible to report some direct statements made by the child, many of the child's communications will be indirect, or made through non-verbal activity and play which will require some interpretive comment: it is a characteristic of play therapy as opposed to investigative work that this should be so.

Whether or not the therapist is called as an expert witness is a matter for the court in which she is appearing, and may depend on her professional qualification or the nature of her position in a particular agency. Whatever her status, however, a therapist giving evidence about therapeutic work undertaken with children is allowed to give evidence of fact and of opinion insofar as this lies within her recognized expertise. (This is in contrast to ordinary witnesses who must confine themselves to factual evidence. Carson, 1990.) It is worth stating that in any case the dichotomy between fact and opinion is nothing like so distinct as the legal profession sometimes appears to maintain, in that any statement about a previous event involves a selective judgement (that is, an opinion) about how it should be described; so that the relationship between the two is perhaps best seen as a continuum rather than as a dichotomy.

This having been said, evidence which appears to fall nearer the factual end of the continuum is likely to carry greater weight in a court setting (among others), in that it has a precision which opinions, being more open to different interpretation, do not have. Evidence which reports what the child said or did without pressure from the therapist thus provides a convincing demonstration of the facts on which the therapist's opinion is based, and the distinction between recorded fact, and inference, hypothesis or opinion is conveyed with greater clarity. Because of the reflective nature of non-directive therapy it is therefore possible to present this form of therapeutic intervention in a manner which carries conviction in a court setting.

Where children are likely to be required to appear as witnesses in criminal proceedings, permission to offer them therapy must be obtained from the Crown Prosecution Service, which has at times (notably in the Crookham Court case) shown a marked reluctance to allow therapeutic work to be undertaken before a trial, on the grounds that this will 'coach' the child and contaminate his evidence. In these circumstances a strong case may be made for non-directive play therapy as the preferred approach, for the reasons given above; that it is largely free from therapist suggestion. The Crown Prosecution Service (CPS) may, however, require that the sessions are video-recorded, a requirement that needs to be treated with some caution (and may indeed be a bar to therapy) especially in cases of children who have been sexually abused and may specifically have been involved in the making of pornographic films.

A further dilemma can arise where the therapist is herself involved in transporting the child to and from the therapy, since if the therapist cannot state that the only contact with the child has been in the therapy sessions, defence lawyers may claim that the child has been coached 'off-stage'. In circumstances where the child is due to appear as a witness, therefore, it is important that the therapist's contact with the child is carefully circumscribed. (See chapter 6 for a further discussion of these issues.)

Finally, in considering the reliability of witness evidence, courts may question the timing of the notes on which the report is based. It is therefore vital that sessions are written up immediately afterwards: stating that notes were written up on the basis of an audio-tape made at the time may be acceptable, but this then may entitle the court to require the tapes to be submitted in evidence (see discussion of immunity from disclosure, chapter 3).

In setting out the report, it is useful to state, briefly and in jargon free language, the orientation adopted in working with the child. Use of the term "therapist" is acceptable where the practitioner has a qualification such as psychotherapist, psychologist or psychiatrist which the courts recognize as an appropriate training for undertaking therapy. Practitioners working from other professional backgrounds, such as social workers, community psychiatric nurses or probation officers, may find it wisest to avoid describing their work as therapy, since the courts appear ready to accept them as experts in counselling, but not therapy. A description such as "direct work, consisting of a non-directive counselling approach which uses play as a medium" seems to be generally acceptable, followed by a brief explanation of the method of working.

Depending on the court's familiarity with therapeutic work, it may be necessary in some circumstances, either in the report or when giving evidence, to clarify the fact that the work was undertaken for therapeutic and not assessment purposes. As we indicate in chapter 1, many settings are unclear about the distinction between the two.

The practitioner's qualifications and experience of working in this way should be stated, and further questions in court, both about training and the method of intervention adopted, should be anticipated. It is regrettably the case that defence lawyers frequently attempt to 'rubbish' the qualifications of social workers and others in related professions in court. These professionals should be careful therefore not to undersell themselves, and to be ready to cite all their qualifications, and training and experience in working with children (not necessarily just that relating to a non-directive approach) when challenged.

In addition to a statement of qualifications, experience and orientation, the report should set out the context of the work, including the number, frequency and length of the therapy sessions, where they took place, the reason for the referral and the problems identified by the referrer.

In his account of work with a boy of nearly four, for example, a social worker reported:

I have been conducting hourly sessions of direct work with James, on an approximately weekly basis, for twenty sessions, in a play room at the X clinic, beginning on October 12th, 1990 and ending on March 21st, 1991. The approach I adopt is non-directive counselling, using play as a medium, in which the child initiates play and conversation while the practitioner attempts to verbalize the child's thoughts and feelings in a non-threatening manner.

I am a qualified social worker, having received the certificate of qualification in social work from ... in ... and I have an honours degree from ... I have undertaken a period of supervised training using this approach while employed by ..., in addition to attending a number of other courses on working with children, and have since used it in my work with children over the past two years.

James was referred to me by the family's social worker, Mr X, who described James's quite severe emotional and physical neglect over a lengthy period of time when he was living at home with his mother and step-father ...

In setting out the work undertaken, it is helpful to anchor this with observations of the child's developmental stage and any particular behavioural or emotional problems which were apparent to the therapist at the outset, giving a factual account of these and the therapist's opinion as to how these might be interpreted, and bearing in mind (as we discuss in chapter 3) that not all problems will have been necessarily apparent at the outset. For example, in the report quoted above, the social worker commented that he seemed immature for his age, especially in his locomotor skills and in his language development, citing the following observations as evidence for this opinion:

When pushing toys along the floor he exhibited the stiff-legged gait normally seen in a toddler, and showed marked hesitancy in climbing stairs. His speech, which was infrequent, was more characteristic of a toddler than of a child of just four, for example "Car, up", when he wanted a toy placed on the table.

Again, social workers need to be careful not to lay themselves open to the charge of appearing to claim expertise in areas where they may be thought not to have it: it is sensible to cite as a comparator observations and experience of working with children of similar ages. The social worker also commented on James's markedly fearful and mistrustful behaviour in the initial sessions, comparing this to what might have been expected from his work with other children and explaining that this was apparent from a reluctance to move from one corner of the playroom, and a great hesitancy when playing with a new toy. The possible interpretations for this behaviour were set out, alongside an opinion that it also could have derived from earlier, damaging experiences. It is useful, where possible, to anticipate these different interpretations, since it is likely that in hostile cross-examination, an attempt will be made to attribute the problematic behaviour to events in the child's immediate circumstances, especially those resulting from the intervention by professionals, rather than to a lack of appropriate care in the setting from which the child has, as in this case, been removed. It is always more convincing to demonstrate that in forming an opinion prior account has been taken of alternative viewpoints. Thus:

This unease was more marked than I would normally expect to find in a child of this age. It may have been due to a number of causes (for example, to not having a familiar adult with him, to having moved home recently, and to having seen a variety of strangers in professional roles over a short period of time.) However, his severe inhibition against exploring the play room, and the way in which he seemed to anticipate from me a strong negative reaction when he did take any initiative, seemed to make it more likely that this stemmed from earlier frightening and punitive experiences rather than arising from anxiety of strangers.

In giving an account of the therapeutic sessions, it is usually best to set out the work in themes, illustrating each of them with a direct, verbatim account of what took place, and showing, again with factual quotation, ways in which the themes may have altered during therapy. It is not, of course, appropriate to give a detailed account of what took place in each session, so it is necessary to select the themes which seem significant in terms of the child's experiences and progress through therapy.

In the case of James, the social worker noted that as James became more trustful of him, his generalized inhibitions were replaced by specific fears, as well as the beginnings of greater assertiveness and naughtiness. He described how these fears, and the process of mastering them, were expressed in James's play:

The specific form his fears took were: fear of being shut in, and fear of the dark; fear of punishment when making a mess; and fear of his own destructiveness ... In the process of mastering his fears, James often played out the theme of something bad happening to a boy [for example, locked in a garage, buried in the sand], and then the boy being rescued and taken to somewhere safe where he was given food and drink. On one occasion, he said, "Mummy shut me in there", and I reflected his feelings about this back to him in terms of this being frightening for him. This theme in his play seemed in my opinion to parallel his earlier experiences with his parents and then the loving care by his foster parents with whom he is currently living.

The report then goes on to describe changes in James's play which occurred during the later stages of therapy, where he enacted scenes of tea parties and bed times, with food being shared among the toys and soft animals, and the animals being tucked up in bed. The social worker interpreted this as evidence of a development in his social skills, and a growing confidence of being loved and looked after.

It is appropriate to highlight any observed changes in behaviour and development at the conclusion of therapy which are noticeable in relation to the observations recorded at the outset: in James's case, his gross motor skills were more appropriate to his chronological age (jumping and running easily), his fine motor skills were developing rapidly (he had begun to draw), and his language, although still sporadic, had also developed in that now he used age-appropriate sentence structures, and was capable of abstract speech.

The report should conclude with a summarizing assessment on how the child now appears, which takes into account his current circumstances and the extent to which they meet his needs, together with any predictive comment about the child's future needs and well-being. Thus the report on James concluded:

He gives every indication of becoming a confident, loving and intelligent boy, and his present environment appears to provide him with the care he lacked previously. He does, however, seem to need extra attention during times of stress, probably as a result of his past experiences. He may be more vulnerable to changes in his current environment than most children and his carers will benefit from extra support in caring for him since it is likely that at times of difficulty, his earlier pattern of fear and timidity may re-emerge.

APPEARING IN COURT

It is beyond the scope of this book to discuss in detail the way in which professionals should present themselves and give evidence in court, and the reader is referred elsewhere for guidance on general issues to do with court processes, responding to cross-examination, and establishing their credibility as witnesses. (See for example, James et al., 1988; Carson, 1990.) We have attempted in the discussion above to highlight some of the areas of difficulty which therapists need to anticipate in relation to preparing the report and giving evidence on it. Some of these especially concern those who come from professional backgrounds which are more likely to be the subject of critical questioning.

We have already alluded to the direction that questioning may take, which can sometimes be pre-empted by the way in which the report is written. There are a number of other dilemmas which can arise, either relating to the way in which the therapist is questioned, or from other expectations of the court. Given these possible pitfalls, it is often helpful, particularly for the inexperienced practitioner, to go through the report with a colleague before a court appearance, trying to anticipate questions and rehearse ways of responding to them.

Much critical cross-examination seems to focus on the nature of therapy and the extent of the direction and suggestions given to the child by the therapist. For example, in relation to the paintings discussed in an earlier section of this chapter, the therapist could have been challenged about having compared the boy's drawing of a school to a church. It would have been important to emphasize that once having made the comment, the therapist did not develop the observation, since it was not picked up by the child.

In relation to the interpretation of the child's play, it is important to try and anticipate, as we have suggested, differing interpretations of the activity. Sometimes interpretations are put forward which one has not anticipated. It is usually as well to indicate a general attitude of willingness to consider alternative views, while maintaining that one's original interpretation still seems well founded (assuming, of course, that it does).

Difficulty will arise if the court considers that the therapist has embarked on therapy with a firm hypothesis as to the aetiology of the child's problems, and has set out, in therapy, to prove this. It is worth, therefore, being alert to any course of questioning designed to suggest that this is so, since the stance taken by a non-directive play therapist must necessarily be open to alternative hypotheses throughout the sessions.

A professional witness, having given evidence, may be asked to comment on other people's observations of the child. It is advisable not to be drawn into this, especially where it may suggest that professionals are in disagreement with each other and, by implication, their evidence is equally flawed. It is therefore prudent for the therapist to stick to commenting on what she has seen and worked with.

After presenting her evidence, the therapist may be asked by the court to continue working with the child. Here, the therapist needs to be alert to the possibility of being required to work in ways which are untherapeutic or seem likely to be counter-productive. One court, for example, sought to make an order for therapy of an abused child to continue, at the same time as allowing the perpetrator to return home. The therapist declined to act, explaining that, in her view, the therapy could not offer the child protection and would be unhelpful and even possibly harmful for the child in such circumstances.

In other situations, where for example criminal proceedings are contemplated, the court may require the therapy to be video recorded. Where, as has happened occasionally, this proves to be traumatizing for the child, the therapist may need to request the court to reconsider the requirement.

In conclusion, it is worth noting that there is an inherent tension in presenting material of a therapeutic nature with its high emotional content in a court setting. Courts are geared towards the scrutiny of so-called 'hard' data and may be unreceptive to the exploration of nuances of feeling and unclear about therapeutic processes. However, the therapist's evidence, and in consequence the child's position is strengthened if it can be shown to be based on good observation; careful recording; clarity of thinking; an understanding of the distinction between fact and hypothesis or interpretation; a lack of bias; and an openness to alternative viewpoints; and above all, a concern for the well-being of the child.

References

Aldgate, J. and Simmonds, J. (eds) (1988) **Direct Work with Children**. Batsford: London.

Alford, C. (1983) **Play Therapy: a Cognitive Approach**. Unpublished dissertation: University of Leicester.

Allen, F.H. (1942) **Psychotherapy with Children**. New York: Norton and Co.

Axline, V. (1946) **Dibs in Search of Self**. New York: Ballantine Books.

Axline, V. (1976) Play Therapy Procedures and Results. In Schaefer, C. (ed.) **The Therapeutic Use of Child's Play**, pp. 209–219. New York: Jason Aronson Inc. [First published in 1955 in the **American Journal of Orthopsychiatry 25**: 618–626.].

Axline, V. (1987) **Play Therapy**. New York: Ballantine Books.

Barker, P. (1988) **Basic Child Psychiatry** (5th edn). Oxford: Blackwell Scientific Publications.

Benton, N. (1991) **Surrounded by Silence: Boys as Victims of Sexual Abuse**. Unpublished dissertation, University of Hull.

Berry, J. (1978) Daily Experience in Residential Care for Children and their Care-givers. In CCETSW Study No 1, **Good Enough Parenting**, pp. 181–192. London: CCETSW.

Betensky, M. (1973) **Self-Discovery Through Self-Expression**. Springfield, IL: CC Thomas.

Bevan, H. (1989) **Child Care Law**. London: Butterworth.

Bixler, R. (1949) Limits are therapy. **Journal of Consulting Psychology 13**: 1–11.

Brent, London Borough of (1985) **A Child in Trust: The Report of the Panel of Inquiry into the Circumstances Surrounding the Death of Jasmine Beckford**. Middlesex: London Borough of Brent.

Browne, K., Davies, C. and Stratton, P. (1988) **Early Prediction and Prevention of Child Abuse**. Chichester: John Wiley and Sons.

Bruner, J.S., Olver, R. and Greenfield, P.M. (eds) (1966) **Studies in Cognitive Growth**. New York: John Wiley.

Butler-Sloss (1988) **Report of the Inquiry into Child Abuse in Cleveland, 1987**. Cm. 412. London: HMSO.

Carson, D. (1990) **Professionals and the Courts: A Handbook for Expert Witnesses**. Birmingham: Venture Press.

Cassirer, E. (1944) **An Essay on Man**. New Haven: Yale University Press.

Cassirer, E. (1955) **The Philosophy of Symbolic Forms**, vol. 2. New Haven: Yale University Press.

Ceci, S.J., Toglia, M.P. and Ross, D.F. (eds) (1987) **Children's Eyewitness Memory**. New York: Springer-Verlag.

Chomsky, N. (1966) **Cartesian Linguistics: A Chapter in the History of National Thought**. New York: Harper & Row.

Clayden, M. (1986) **Child's Play: Communication and Therapy within a Social Work Context**. University of Leicester: unpublished dissertation.

Corsini, R.J. (1966) **Roleplaying in Psychotherapy. A Manual**. Chicago: Aldine.

Dicks, H. (1967) **Marital Tensions**. London: Tavistock.

Dockar-Drysdale, B. (1970) **Therapy in Child Care**. London: Longman.

Dorfman, E. (1976) Play Therapy. In Rogers, C. (ed.) **Client Centred Therapy**, pp. 235–278. London: Constable.

Doyle, C. (1990) **Working with Abused Children**. Hampshire: Macmillan Education.

Ekman, P. (1989) **Why Kids Lie**. New York: Viking Penguin.

Ekstein, R. (1966) **Children of Time and Space, of Action and Impulse**. New York: Meredith.

Erikson, E.H. (1963) **Childhood and Society**. New York: Norton and Co.

Erikson, E.H. (1964) **Insight and Responsibility**. New York: Norton and Co.

Erikson, E.H. (1968) **Identity, Youth and Crisis**. New York: Norton and Co.

Erikson, E.H. (1977) **Toys and Reasons**. New York: Norton and Co.

Fairbairn, W. (1954) **Object Relations Theory of the Personality**. New York: Basic Books.

Finkelhor, D., Araji, S., Baron, L., Browne, A., Peters, S. and Wyatt, G. (1986) **A Sourcebook on Child Sexual Abuse**. London; New York: Sage Publications.

Flavell, J.H., Botkin, P.T., Fry, C.L., Wright, J.W. and Jarvis, P.E. (1968) **The Development of Role-taking and Communication Skills in Children**. New York: Wiley.

Flavell, J.H. (1985) **Cognitive Development**. Englewood Cliffs, NJ: Prentice-Hall.

Fraser, S. (1989) **My Father's House, a Memoir of Incest and Healing**. London: Virago Press.

Freud, S. (1900) **The Interpretation of Dreams** (1965 edn). New York: Hearst.

Freud, S. (1974) In Strachey, J. (ed.) **The Complete Psychological Works**. London: Hogarth Press.

Frosh, S. (1987) Issues for Men Working with Sexually Abused Children. **British Journal of Psychotherapy 3**: 332–339.

Furniss, T. (1991) **Multi-Professional Handbook of Child Sexual Abuse**. London: Routledge.

Gagnon, J.H. (1972) **The Creation of the Sexual in Early Adolescence**. New York: Norton.

Giaretto, H. (1982) **Integrated Treatment of Child Sexual Abuse**. Palo Alto, California: Science and Behaviour Books.

Gill, M.M. (1967) The Primary Process. In Holt, R.R. (ed.) Motives and Thought: Psychoanalytic Essays in Honor of David Rapaport. **Psychological Issues V** (2–3): Mono. 18–19.

Glaser, D. and Frosh, S. (1988) **Child Sexual Abuse**. London: Macmillan Education.

Gomez-Schwartz, Horowitz, J. and Cardarelli, A. (1990) **Child Sexual Abuse: The Initial Effects**. London: Sage Publications.

Hall, C.S. and Lindzey, G. (1978) **Theories of Personality**. Chichester: John Wiley and Sons.

Harris, P.L. (1989) **Children and Emotion**. Oxford: Basil Blackwell.

Harter, S. (1977) A Cognitive-Developmental Approach to Children's Expression of Conflicting Feelings and a Technique to Facilitate Such Expression in Play Therapy. **Journal of Consulting and Clinical Psychology 45**: 417–432.

Haugaard, J. and Reppucci, N.D. (1988) **The Sexual Abuse of Children**. San Francisco: Jossey-Bass.

Hickmann, M. (1986) Psychosocial Aspects of Language Acquisition. In Fletcher, P., Garman, M. (eds) **Language Acquisition: Studies in First Language Development** (2nd edn). Cambridge: Cambridge University Press.

Horowitz, J., Gomes-Schwartz, B. and Cardavelli, A. (1990) **Child Sexual Abuse, The Initial Effects**. London; New York: Sage Publications.

Huizinga, J. (1949) **Homo Ludens**. London: Routledge and Kegan Paul.

Isaacs, S. (1933) **Social Development in Young Children**. London: Routledge.

James, A. and Wilson, K. (1991) Marriage, social policy and social work. **Journal of Social Work Practice 5**: 169–178.

James, A., Wilson, K. and Parry, M. (eds) (1988) **Social Work in Family Proceedings: a Practice Guide**. London: Routledge.

Jehu, D., Gazan, D. and Klassen, C. (1989) **Beyond Sexual Abuse**. London: John Wiley and Sons.

Jones, D.P.H. and Krugman, R. (1986) Can a Three-Year-Old Child Bear Witness to her Assault and Attempted Murder? **Journal of Child Abuse and Neglect 10**: 253–258.

Jones, D.P.H. and McQuiston, M. (1985) **Interviewing the Sexually Abused Child**. London: Gaskell.

Kagan, J. and Coles, R. (1972) **Twelve to Sixteen: Early Adolescence**. New York: Norton.

Kezur, B. (1981) Play Therapy as a Mode of Treatment for Disturbed Children. In Martel, S. (ed.) **Direct Work with Children**. London: Bedford Square Press.

Kroger, J. (1989) **Identity in Adolescence**. London: Routledge.

Laing, R. (1961) **The Self and Others**. London: Tavistock Publications.

Laishley, J. (1983) **Working With Young Children**. London: Edward Arnold.

Lee, P.R., Ornstein, R.E., Galin, D., Deikman, A. and Tart, C.T. (eds) (1976) **Symposium on Consciousness**. New York: Viking Press.

Lenneberg, E.H. (1967) **Biological Foundations of Language**. New York: Wiley.

Levy, D. (1938) Release Therapy in Young Children. **Psychiatry 1**: 387–389.

Lowenfeld, M. (1979) **The World Technique**. London: Allen and Unwin.

Marvasti, J. (1989) Play Therapy with Sexually Abused Children. In Sgroi, S. (ed.) **Vulnerable Populations**, pp. 1–41. Massachusetts: Lexington Books.

Mattinson, J. and Sinclair, I. (1979) **Mate and Stalemate: Working with Marital Problems in a Social Services Department**. Oxford: Basil Blackwell.

Mearns, D. and Thorne, B. (1990) **Person-centred Counselling in Action**. London: Sage Publications.

Miller, H.E. (1948) Play Therapy for the Institutional Child. **Nervous Child 7**: 311–312.

Moustakas, C. (1953) **Children in Play Therapy**. New York: McGraw Hill.

Moustakas, C. (1959) **Psychotherapy with Children: The Living Relationship**. New York: Harper & Row.

Moustakas, C. and Schalock, H.D. (1955) An Analysis of Therapist Child Interaction in Play Therapy. **Child Development 26** (2): 143–157.

Mussen, P.H., Conger, J.J., Kagan, J. and Huston, A.C. (1990) **Child Development and Personality** (7th edn). London: Harper & Row.

Neusner, J. (1981) Peter. In Martel, S. (ed.) **Direct Work with Children**. London: Bedford Square Press.

Newson, E. (in press) The Barefoot Play Therapist. In Lane, D. and Miller, A., **The Handbook of Child and Adolescent Therapy**. Milton Keynes: Open University Press.

Newson, J. and Newson, E. (1979) **Toys and Playthings**. London: Allen and Unwin.

Oaklander, V. (1978) **Windows to our Children**. New York: Real People Press.

Owen, P. and Curtis, P. (1983) **Techniques for Working With Children**. Owen and Curtis.

Petersen, A.C. (1988) Adolescent Development. **Annual Review of Psychology 39**: 583–607.

Piaget, J. (1952) **The Origins of Intelligence in Children**. New York: Norton.

Piaget, J. (1962) **Play, Dreams and Imitation in Childhood**. New York: Norton.

Piaget, J. (1965) **The Moral Judgment of the Child**. New York: Free Press.

Piaget, J. (1967) **Six Psychological Studies**. New York: Random House.

Piaget, J. and Inhelder, B. (1969) **Mental Imagery in the Child**. New York: Basic Books.

Pynoos, R. and Eth, S. (1984) The Child as Witness to Homicide. **Journal of Social Issues 40**: 87–108.

Pynoos, R. and Eth, S. (1986) Witness to Violence: The Child Interview. **Journal of the American Academy of Child Psychiatry 25** (3): 306–319.

Rado, S. (1969) **Adaptation of Psychodynamics: Motivation and Control**. New York: Science House.

Redgrave, K. (1987) **Child's Play**. Cheshire: Boys' and Girls' Welfare Society.

Reisman, J. (1973) **Principles of Psychotherapy with Children**. New York: John Wiley and Sons.

Report of the Advisory Group on Video Evidence (1989). London: HMSO.

Richardson, A. (1969) **Mental Imagery**. London: Routledge and Kegan Paul.

Rogers, C. (1976) **Client-Centred Therapy** (1976 edn). London: Constable.

Rogers, N.S. et al. (1989) **Child Abuse and Neglect. Facing the Challenge**. Milton Keynes: Batsford Ltd and Open University.

Ross, A.O. (1959) **The Practice of Clinical Child Psychology**. New York: Grune and Stratton.

Saint-Exupéry, A. de (1943) **The Little Prince**. New York: Harcourt, Brace and World.

Salter, A.C. (1988) **Treating Child Sex Offenders and Victims**. Sage Publishing.

Sapir, E. (1958) **Culture, Language and Personality: Selected Essays**. Berkeley, CA: University of California Press.

Satir, V. (1967) **Conjoint Family Therapy**. Palo Alto, CA: Science and Behavior Books.

Schachtel, E. (1959) **Metamorphosis**. New York: Basic Books.

Schaefer, C. (1976) **The Therapeutic Use of Children's Play**. New York: Jason Aronson Inc.

Sgroi, S. (1988) **Clinical Intervention in Child Sexual Abuse**. Massachusetts: Lexington Books.

Sgroi, S (1989) **Vulnerable Populations: Sexual Abuse Treatment for Children, Adult**

Survivors, Offenders, and Persons with Mental Retardation. Massachusetts: Lexington Books.

Sheldon, B. (1983) The Use of Single Case Experimental Designs in the Evaluation of Social Work. **British Journal of Social Work 13** (5).

Singer, J. (1966) **Daydreaming: an Introduction to the Experimental Study of Inner Experience**. New York: Random House.

Snow, C.E. (1986) Conversations with Children. In Fletcher, P. and Garman, M. (eds) **Language Acquisition: Studies in First Language Development** (2nd edn). Cambridge: Cambridge University Press.

Solomon, J. (1938) Active Play Therapy. **Journal of Orthopsychiatry 8**: 479–498.

Stern, D.N. (1985) **The Interpersonal World of the Infant**. New York: Basic Books.

Stevens, C. and Walsh, E. (1987) **Family Law Reports**, Special Issue no. 4. London: Jordan and Sons.

Sutton, C. (1979) **Psychology for Social Workers and Counsellors**. London: Routledge and Kegan Paul.

Taft, J. (1933) **The Dynamics of Therapy in a Controlled Relationship**. New York: Macmillan.

Tinbergen, N. and Tinbergen, E. (1983) **'Autistic' Children**. London: Allen and Unwin.

Truax, C. and Carkhuff, R. (1967) **Toward Effective Counselling and Psychotherapy**. Chicago: Aldine.

Vygotsky, L.S. (1962) **Thought and Language**. Cambridge, MA: MIT Press.

Walls, V. (1972) A Theoretical Study of Daydreaming Activity. University of Texas at Austin: unpublished.

Wellman, H. (1990) **The Child's Theory of Mind**. London; Cambridge, MA: MIT Press.

Werner, H. (1948) **Comparative Psychology of Mental Development**. New York: International Universities Press.

Werner, H. and Kaplan, B. (1963) **Symbol Formation**. New York: John Wiley.

Whitaker, D. (1985) **Using Groups to Help People**. London: Routledge.

Whorf, B.L. (1956) **Language, Thought and Reality**. Cambridge, MA: MIT Press.

Williamson, K. (1990) **Communicating with Children**. Available from the author, Grimsby College, Grimsby, North Humberside.

Wilson, K. and James, A. (1991) Research in Therapy with Couples: an Overview. In Hooper, D. and Dryden, W. (eds) **Couple Therapy: a Handbook**, pp. 270–294. Milton Keynes: Open University Press.

Winnicott, D.W. (1988) **Playing and Reality** (1986 edn). London: Pelican Books.

Wolff, S. (1986) Childhood Psychotherapy. In Bloch, S. (ed.) **An Introduction to the Psychotherapies** (2nd edn). Oxford: Oxford University Press.

Wolff, S. (1989) **Childhood and Human Nature**. London: Routledge.

Wyre, R. and Smith, A. (1990) **Women, Men and Rape**. London: Headway, Hodder and Stoughton.

———— Index ————

Note. Sub-entries are in alphabetical order, except where chronological order is more useful.

guns and weapons, toy 83, 86

historical perspective 16–21
homicide witnesses 37, 42, 152
hospitalization 35
hypnotic toys 55

identity *see* roles
identity versus role confusion stage 136,
    150–8
    and sexual abuse 167–8
imagery *see* mental imagery
imitation 38
inadequacy feelings of therapist 148
independence
    false, stage of 111–14
    see also autonomy
industry versus inferiority stage 136,
    143–9, 155
    and sexual abuse 166–7
inferiority *see* industry
information *see* confidentiality; disclosure;
    family and primary carers
initial sessions *see* first sessions
initiative
    and mutuality in case study of process
        of play therapy 114–18
    versus guilt stage 136, 141–2, 155
    and sexual abuse 165–6
inner speech 44–5, 48, 53
inner symbolic representations *see* inner
    speech; mental imagery
inquiries, public 2–3, 94, 169, 211, 212,
    216
insurance for child, therapist's
    involvement as 71
intelligent action 38
interpretive approach 6–7
    avoiding *see* non-directive play therapy
intrusiveness 190–1, 197–8
issues and themes
    personal 74–5
    planning 73–6
    sexually abused child, therapy for 174,
        187–8
    see also practice skills and issues

joy of self-expression 27, 33, 47, 49,
    56

labelling 154–5
language
    and case study of process 110, 116
    and feelings 45
    inner speech 44–5, 48, 53
    and mental activity 43–4
    and mental imagery 45–6
    and symbolic play 43–7, 53–4, 56, 58
    of therapist *see* reflection
limits *see* boundaries
listening and attending 24–5
loss 177
loss and separation 67, 68, 72
    see also displacement; trauma

meaningfulness 40, 53
medical examination of abused child 169
memory and memories 41–2, 48, 54, 56,
    153
    loss 37, 183, 185–6
mental activity and language 43–4
mental activity represented by symbols 40
mental development
    and symbolic play *see* symbolic play
    see also cognitive; thought
mental imagery 40–4, 48, 50
    and language 45–6
mess 115–16, 117–18, 204, 206
middle childhood: emotional
    development 143–9
middle sessions in case study of process of
    play therapy 111–14, 127–8
mirroring *see* reflection
mistrust *see* trust versus mistrust stage
monitoring therapy 99–100
mothers *see* family and primary carers
motor schemas 34–5, 37, 39, 45, 184
murder *see* homicide witnesses
mutuality and initiative 114–18

non-conservation 46
non-directive play therapy 2, 16–30
    historical perspective 16–21
    principles and practice 21–30
    see also emotional development;
        planning; practice skills and issues;
        process; sexually abused child,
        therapy for; symbolic play
non-interpretive work *see* non-directive

non-possessive warmth, need for 22
non-verbal communication 128
  see also body language; eye contact;
    personal space
normal play 121–4
notes *see* written records

obesity 186
object relations therapy 6–7, 17
objective schemas 34–5, 39
organization of schema 39
organized activities 49, 143–4, 146
Orkneys 215, 218
outer symbolic representations 48

paediatrician 169
painting and drawing 192, 197, 199–200,
    215
  and case study of process 112, 114–15
  and sexually abused child, therapy for
    201–3
  and symbolic play 35, 50, 51, 54–5, 59
past experiences reintegrated 55–7
patience 111
peer groups and friendships 143–4, 145,
    153, 166, 201
permissive therapy *see* non-directive play
    therapy
personal feelings *see* emotional
    development; feelings and
    emotions *and under* therapist
personal issues *see* issues
personal schemas and symbolic play
    34–5, 36, 39
personal space
  eye contact 127–8
  and sexually abused child 173–5
  ignorance of boundaries 29, 104,
    105, 177–9
physical appearance and clothes 122,
    130, 145, 186–7
physical contact 29
physical setting *see* setting
Pigot Report 212
planning decisions and tasks 65–102
  initial 66–76
  further 76–102
  need for individual therapy 66–70
  referral and referring agency 71–3

and sexually abused child, therapy
    for 170–1
  therapist, issues for 73–6
play
  diagnosis and assessment 13–14
  functions of 46–50
  see also non-directive play therapy
playdough *see* clay and playdough
play-related interventions 11–14
  communications 12–13, 15
pornographic films 94, 172, 219
post-traumatic amnesia 37
practice skills and issues 189–224
  court setting 218–24
  disclosure and validation 210–17
  establishing limits 205–10
  guidelines 23
  reflection 189–205
  and sexually abused child, therapy for
    201–3, 210–14, 217
praise 147–8
preparatory work 97–9
primary carers *see* family and primary
    carers
privacy 195, 200
  and planning 81–2, 92
  see also confidentiality
process of play therapy 103–34
  example *see* case study of process
  recording 95
psychic reality 13
psycho-analytic play therapy 5–6, 15
psychotherapy, different approaches to
    4–16
  abreactive play therapy 9–10, 15
  cognitive-behavioural approaches 7–8,
    15
  commonalities in 14–16
  object relations therapy 6–7
  play-related interventions 11–14, 15
  psycho-analytic play therapy 5–6, 15
  release therapy 8–9, 15
  structured/focused play therapy 10–11
  see also non-directive play therapy
puberty 151
  see also adolescence
public inquiries 2–3, 94, 169, 211, 212,
    216
puppets 14

feelings expressed or experienced 174–7

issues and themes 174

and planning 66, 68, 69, 71–2, 75, 77, 94, 170–1

referral 172

self-mutilation 179–83

sexualized behaviour 29, 104, 105, 177–9

and skills and issues 201–3, 210–14, 217

and symbolic play 37, 51, 60

symptomology of 169–70

therapist, issues for 187–8

timing 172–3

see also court proceedings

shame *see* autonomy versus shame and doubt stage; guilt

shyness 144, 153

size of room 80

skills and issues *see* practice skills and issues

sleeping problems of sexually abused 186–7

social games *see* organized activities

soundproofing 80–1

space, personal *see* personal space

speech *see* language

squiggle game 7

story-telling, mutual 10–11

structuring 24

structured exercises 50, 57–9

structured play therapy 10–11

submission 183

sucking *see* bottle, baby's

supervision of therapist 97

symbolic play and mental development 13, 31–64

activities 50–5

adaptation and assimilation 32–3

and case study of process of play therapy 118–20, 126–7

consciousness and mental development 36

coping mechanisms and conscious awareness 36–40

language and mental activity 43–4

mental imagery 40–3

and language 45–6

organization based on schemes 33–4

past experiences reintegrated 55–7

personal and objective schemas 34–5

and sexually abused child, therapy for 175–6, 178–9, 184

structured exercises 57–9

thinking in mental images 42–3

toys and play materials as early symbolizations of thought 47

utilization of 50–5

see also role playing

symptomology of sexually abused child, therapy for 169–70

synthesis 42, 48

see also condensation

taping *see* audio-taping; vehicles, play

tea service, toy 86

teaching and parenting role, avoiding 191–2

tentative nature of reflection 26

tentative reflection 26

therapist

assessment of 99–100

commitment 73–4

competence, sense of 147

feelings 53, 63

awareness of 28–31

and case study of process 111, 132–3

guilt 132–3

inadequacy 148

gender 74, 188

issues for 73–6, 187–8

language *see* reflection

limitations 132–3

as onlooker 127

personal characteristics needed 22–3

personal issues 74–5

and planning 74, 81–2, 99–100

recording work *see* records

relationship with 53

resilience 63

setting 74

sexual arousal 187, 188

statement 75–6

supervision of 97, 187

and symbolic play 53, 63

see also emotional development; planning; practice skills and issues;